D0437851

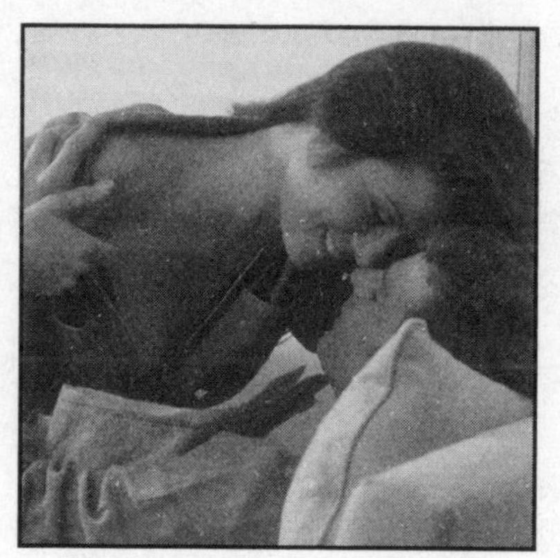

THE 10 SECRETS TO GREAT SEX

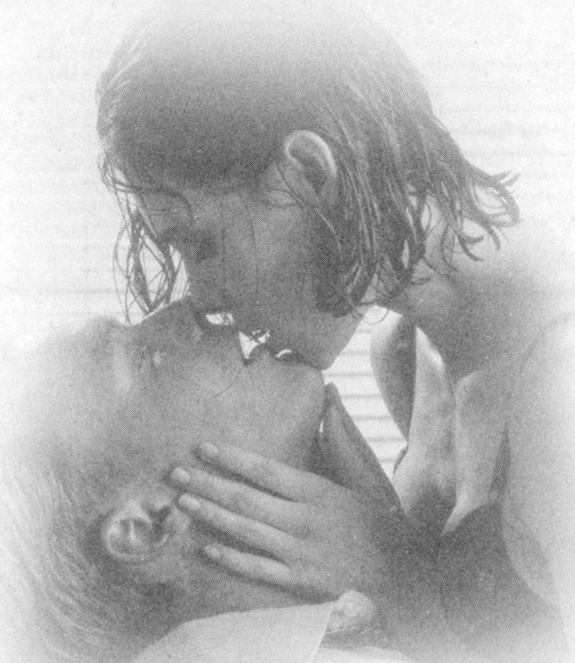

THE 10 SECRETS TO GREAT SEX

BY FELICIA ZOPOL AND

THE SINCLAIR INTIMACY INSTITUTE

RUNNING PRESS
PHILADELPHIA • LONDON

Printed in the United States

Digit on the right indicates the number of this printing

Library of Congress Cataloging-in-Publication Number 2002100444

ISBN 0-7624-1154-6

Cover and Interior design: Gwen Galeone
Editor: Deborah Grandinetti
Sinclair Intimacy Institute Editor: Susan Yeager Montani
Photographs supplied by the Sinclair Intimacy Institute
Typography: Dante, Schneidler, Universe.

This book may be ordered by mail from the publisher.
Please include $2.50 for postage and handling.
But try your bookstore first!

Running Press Book Publishers
125 South Twenty-second Street
Philadelphia, Pennsylvania 19103-4399

TABLE OF CONTENTS

TABLE OF CONTENTS

INTRODUCTION:
A Letter from the Sinclair Intimacy Institute

Dear Reader,

Perhaps you've seen our ads in your favorite magazines. They're the ones that feature photographs of attractive couples in a loving embrace. Typically—although not always—the headline reads something like: "Great Lovers Are Made, Not Born," or "Sex Education for Me? Know-How Is Still the Best Aphrodisiac."

Those ads are for our top-selling programs, including the Better Sex Video Series®, which we at the Sinclair Intimacy Institute have produced in cooperation with leading sex educators, family and marriage counselors, and therapists. Our intent has always been to provide explicit—and tasteful—sex education for committed couples. We believe there's a real need for accurate sexual health information, and our sales have proven us right. The Better Sex Video Series® is the best-selling sex education video series in the United States, selling more than four million videos in over twenty-four countries since we launched the line in 1991. Our library now includes more than fifty titles. We also produce a line of sexually oriented toys and sexual-health related products.

Why provide sexual education for couples? Haven't most adults figured it out for themselves? Sadly, no. Countless therapists tell us that much of their job is providing accurate sexual information and clarifying misinformation, which is the cause of many sexual conflicts.

Consider the fact that lovemaking skills aren't formally taught, the way, say, driving skills are. Anyone who wants a driver's license has to learn the rules of the road, and prove competence on both a written and practical test. But when it comes to sexual intimacy, people are pretty much left to fend for themselves. Just think back to your own sources of sex information. The lack of sex education and the amount of misinformation are unfortunate, given the power of a mutually satisfying intimate relationship to enhance the lives of both partners. Accurate sex information can certainly sweeten any relationship and help it endure.

The 10 Secrets to Great Sex is our first book. It distills the wisdom in our videos, in a form that may be more accessible for couples who prefer to learn through the written word. We hope that this book stimulates discussion between you and your partner, and helps improve every aspect of your intimate relationship. (Good communication is an essential ingredient in a satisfying intimate relationship.) In our effort to be as complete as possible, we will no doubt cover ground already familiar to you. But we do hope to provide you with several new tips that will intrigue you enough to try them. Share what you've discovered with the one you love . . . and celebrate a whole new world of sexual intimacy and sensual excitement!

Sincerely,

Susan Yeager Montani, Project Editor
on behalf of the staff at the Sinclair Intimacy Institute

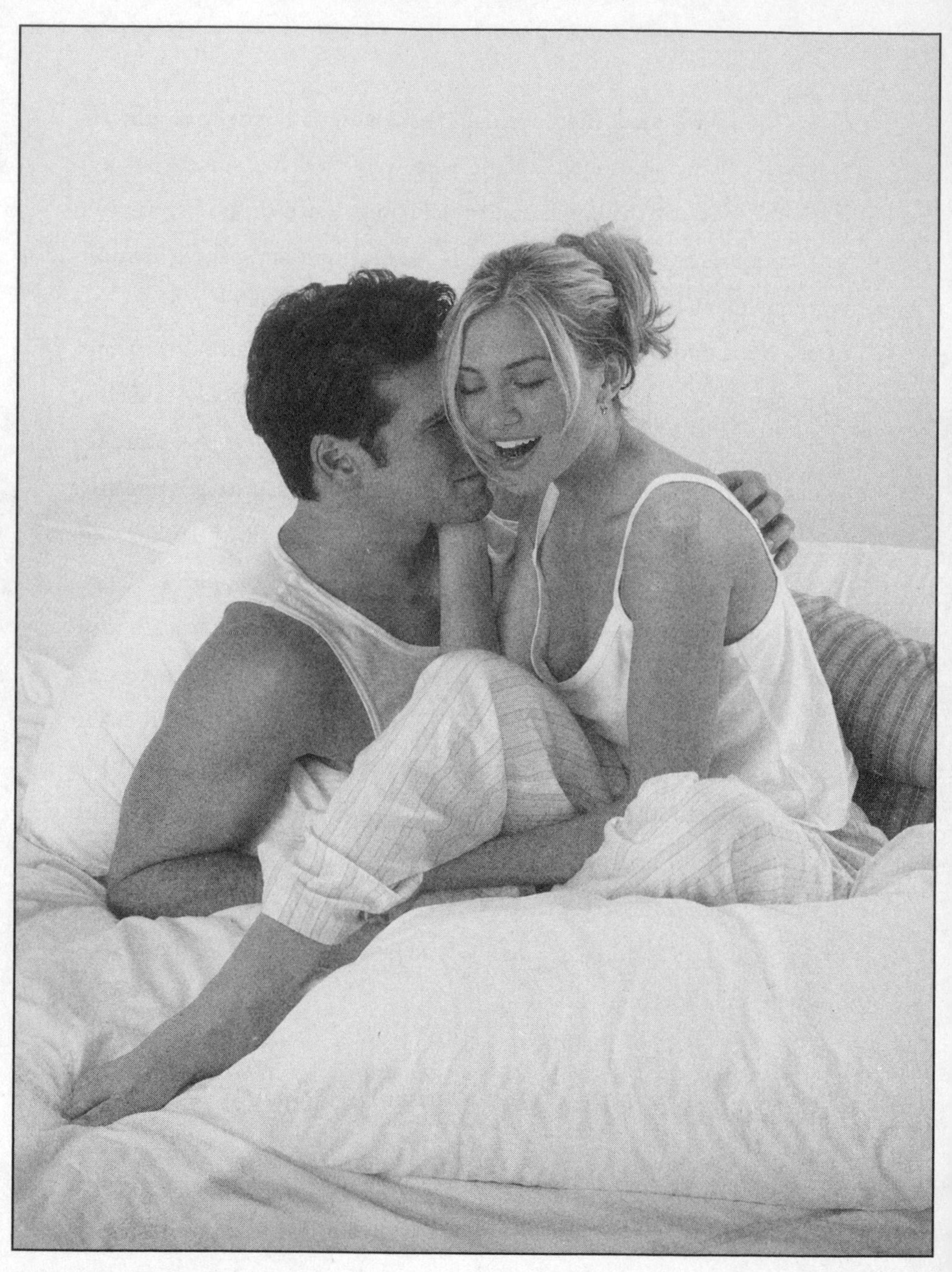

SECRET #1

Make the Decision to Go for It!

> *. . . lifelong committed sex has the potential to be more thrilling, more varied, more satisfying in every way than any other sexual arrangement you can think of.*
>
> —DAGMAR O'CONNOR
> *How to Make Love to the Same Person for the Rest of Your Life*

We are built for pleasure. Make no mistake about it. Anyone intimate with human anatomy can give you plenty of evidence. Why else would our nervous system, muscles and bones be wrapped in a large, soft, sensory organ—the skin—which is exquisitely capable of registering not only sensations of touch, but also pressure and temperature? Why else would there be so many receptors just beneath the skin's surface, particularly in the fingers, lips, genitals and palm of the hand? Or nerve pathways capable of triggering impulses to the brain when these erogenous zones are stimulated?

Why else would we be gifted with a nervous system and sense organs so interconnected that the mere sight of a lover, or the sound of a lover's voice, can bring a flush of warmth between the legs? Why else would we come equipped with erectile tissue—yes, it's there in women, too, in the clitoris and nipples—capable of engorging with blood and then emptying in an ecstatic, body-thrilling rush?

It's curious, isn't it—given all the pleasure pathways bequeathed to us at birth—that we aren't walking around in a constant state of pleasure. In a world where everything seeks after its pleasure, where the hummingbird drinks the nectar of the flower, and the cat seeks out warm, sunny nooks to nap, you would think human couples could easily find their bliss, too. After all, it seems like such a perfect pairing: the male and female sexual organs are designed expressly to fit, excite and satiate the other. And the hearts and minds of man and woman are uniquely endowed to elevate this essentially animal act into a sublimely satisfying experience of soul communion.

So why does the passion rarely seem to last? Why are so many "pleasure partners" unsuccessful at cultivating their garden of delights, or making it more lush as the years go on?

There are probably as many reasons as there are unfulfilled couples. But there are certain problems that marriage and family therapists see again and again. One, mentioned earlier, is that couples lack accurate and precise information about their own sexuality, and/or their partner's, as well as the attitudes, skills and techniques that bring fulfillment. So they venture into their intimate relations without much skill or enthusiasm, naively expecting everything to go right. This half-hearted approach, in and of itself, indicates that something has already gone wrong in the relationship. Healthy couples seek to learn and grow together. Those who aren't willing to risk doing some things differently to make their intimate life better are likely to continue to drift apart, rather than grow more deeply in love.

Lack of information is easily remedied. That's why we've written *The 10 Secrets to Great Sex*. You'll find information demystifying the male and female erogenous zones in Chapter 4, plus more technical advice on how to use sexual positions for maximum pleasure in Chapter 5. Chapter 6 takes you step-by-step into the realms of multiple and "G-spot" orgasms. Chapter 10 provides explicit advice about how to pleasure a partner orally and anally. Chapters 7, 8 and 9 explore ways that you can bring variety and newness to your intimate time together. Mastering this material will give you the makings of a great lover.

But technical know-how isn't enough. We believe that great sex is more than just physical—it also has to engage your emotions, intellect and spirit. That's why the chapters ahead also address each of these aspects of your relationship. If you aren't relating well at these levels, it can interfere with your sexual relationship. That's why resolving problems within yourself, or between the two of you, in any of these other areas can open the way for the most fulfilling sexual encounters of your life. Couples who work through problems together grow in trust. They have a deeper well of intimacy to draw from. The deepening of trust allows both individuals to completely relax with each other, to be vulnerable and open, two prerequisites for deeply satisfying sex.

What's Putting the Damper on Your Fire?

If you sense there could be more to your sexual life together—more sizzle, more intimacy, more pleasure, more fulfillment—and you aren't sure what is standing in the way, read this next section together. It could help you identify the particular obstacles that have been preventing you and your partner from reaching your sexual potential together. Zeroing in on the problem is powerful, because in naming it, the solution usually becomes apparent. If you are willing to explore this with each other, you're well on your way to a revitalized sexual life. It doesn't matter how long you've been together or how discouraged you've become. Know that if the two of you truly want to reignite this aspect of your lives, you can. It is possible to grow through adversity and become happier and more sexually fulfilled with each other.

Here are common ways couples unwittingly cork the passion:

Passion-Stopper #1: Relegating Intimate Time to the Bottom of Your List

Most romantic partners enjoy an active sex life early in their relationships. But the emphasis on physical passion often gives way to the pressure of everyday responsibilities. Long, soulful talks are replaced with conversations centering on domestic responsibilities, financial concerns, work pressures, the children's needs. Couples with so much on their plates often relegate sex to the bottom of their list of priorities. No wonder that researchers, who wanted to know if there was any basis to the "7-year-itch," found that 75 percent of couples who had been together for seven years said they were dissatisfied with their sex lives and considering an affair.

TIP: *Some people think that extraordinary sex can only happen if the relationship is flawless. Yet couples with disagreements and differences and everyday stress can learn to separate their problems to make room for passion. Sometimes problems need to be temporarily put on hold to replenish your intimacy. The problems will seem easier to address if you've tasted the closeness of your relationship.*

If you want to keep things hot between the two of you, you have to put your relationship at the top of the list. Make intimate time a priority. You may have to take time away from other activities, but consider it time well spent. Realize that the pleasure you share in your intimate time together will spill into every other area of your life. You will find that mutually fulfilling physical intimacy forges a "pleasure bond," which makes it easier to disregard the small annoyances that are inevitable when two people live together. It will also keep you vital, giving you more "juice" to bring to your children, your work, or your other affairs in the world. Sexual closeness is the body's emotional fuel. Without it, we run out of gas and our relationship may feel very empty.

Passion-Stopper #2: Assuming You Know What Your Lover Wants

Decide right now that you will no longer assume you know what your partner wants or needs to feel sexually satisfied. Be humble enough to ask. It is naïve to assume the other wants exactly what you want. That's true with regard to the frequency with which you make love, the hour of the day, the level of lighting, the amount of foreplay. And it goes double for something as intimate as manual or oral stimulation. Just because a certain kind of touch, pressure, or speed feels good on your genitals doesn't mean it will bring your partner bliss. Don't be afraid to ask and to keep learning.

Tip: *Watching sex education videos together can pave the way for discussions about sex. The videos often raise issues that partners are afraid to bring up on their own, or did not realize were affecting their relationship. Videos offer assurance that you're not the only ones experiencing difficulties, making the problems less embarrassing and easier to discuss. A good video can also provide positive role models and may inspire you and your partner to try a new approach to seduction or lovemaking that appeals to you. For more information on different styles of videos, see page 131 in Secret #7, "Make Sex Fun with Toys."*

Passion-Stopper #3: Doing the Same Things in the Same Way

People grow and change throughout their lives. So don't assume that you or your partner require the same approach to sex or the same kind of stimulation today as you did earlier in the relationship. If schedules have changed at work, or you've had a child together, you may need to approach your intimate life in a new way.

This made all the difference for Rodney and Michelle. They had a wonderful sexual life before Michelle gave birth to their first child. But then things changed. When Michelle was breastfeeding, she lost much of her desire for sex. The demands of childcare left her with little energy. When she did have intercourse with Rodney, it was painful. Her vagina had not yet healed from the birth. Nor did it produce the same amount of lubrication as before.

At first, Rodney tried to accommodate her by doing without sex. But then he grew resentful. When they talked about what they could do to make things better for both of them, they realized there were alternatives. Now, Rodney takes the time to help his wife relax by giving her an intimate massage or pleasuring her in other ways. They apply lubrication to his penis and her vagina as part of foreplay.

Michelle expresses her love by manually stimulating Rodney's penis. Then she takes charge of her own pleasure, by stroking her vulva with his penis. When she feels ready for intercourse, she puts Rodney's penis all the way in, and moves in ways that feel good to her. By controlling the action, she ensures that intercourse is not painful. These are the changes they have made to make sex good for both of them at this particular stage of their lives.

Stephen and Nancy also found ways to reignite the passion after having a child. Nancy was also exhausted caring for her newborn. A marriage and family counselor recommended that Stephen take on some of the baby's night feeding shifts so Nancy could get the sleep she needed to feel like a whole person again. That helped give Nancy the energy for sex. The couple even hired a babysitter from time to time, so they could focus entirely on each other.

Once Nancy had a little time for herself, she realized that she still liked sex but wanted to put more of an emphasis on pampering when they were intimate. Stephen obliges her by giving her an erotic massage, and by spending more time on foreplay.

"I learned that sex doesn't always have to mean intercourse," says Stephen. "There are many, many ways of sharing pleasure with each other, even when you're tired."

Nancy was thrilled with Stephen's expanded sensual repertoire. "Sex has become a great way to relax, and recharge," says Nancy. "We feel like it makes time for us because it leaves us feeling so happy and energized."

Passion-Stopper #4: Using Sex as a Substitute

Never use sex to make up for lack in some other area of your life. That's putting a burden on your sex life that shouldn't be there. It's much healthier to approach your intimate time together as a celebration of your love and friendship, and of your sexual aliveness.

Sex can become ho hum in an otherwise good relationship when one or both partners stops growing. That's because sexual energy is an expression of the life force. If you are not actively pursuing your goals and dreams, you're pushing down your aliveness. That means you have less of it to bring to the relationship. The extent to which you "sit" on this forward-moving energy in your life—whether it's out of fear, laziness or feelings of unworthiness—is the extent to which you limit the potential for fulfillment within your intimate relationship.

Even the best sex is no substitute for the deep satisfaction that comes when you pursue those things that make you happy—whether that's a hobby, striking out in a new career, or fulfilling a mission that's meaningful to you.

So follow your bliss. And encourage your partner to do the same. Individuals who happily pursue their bliss are naturally magnetic. They have more "juice" in and out of bed. They also tend to be happier in their committed relationships.

This is more than just speculation. A study conducted by the State University of New York at Buffalo found that self-confident people were happier in their marriages. People who were bothered by self-doubt were less satisfied with their relationships, which led them to find greater fault with their partners and back off from them emotionally. And what is it that builds confidence? Taking constructive action to pursue your private passions and realize your dreams.

Passion-Stopper #5: Using Sex as a Weapon

By the same token, sex should never become a weapon. Emotionally mature lovers don't withhold sex as a form of punishment. They open up when they are upset, and talk the problem through. That's not to say you should force yourself to accommodate your partner sexually if you are still deeply upset. But be honest. Give your lover a chance to help you over your upset. Doing so may bring your relationship to an even deeper level of intimacy and mutual satisfaction.

Passion-Stopper #6: Getting Lax About Considerate Behavior

One reason couples enjoy each other's company so much early in the relationship is because they tend to be on their best behavior. The desire to win the affections of the other leads them to be extra considerate, and to give to each other in ways they may not give later. The man may start off bringing flowers to the woman who catches his eye; the woman may bake something special for her man, or spend an hour lovingly massaging his shoulders.

During this initial phase of passion, new couples spend a lot of time touching, holding hands, cuddling and kissing. They regularly express their attraction—both verbally and physically. They tend to engage in long discussions, talking about their deepest feelings and interests, and listening intently to one another.

Is it any wonder the sex is so good?

As time goes on, one or both individuals may start to take the other for granted. They may stop doing the little things that so endeared the other. Expressions of affection may grow less frequent, as criticism and disagreements grow more frequent. They may neglect those long soulful conversations, saving their talk for divvying up chores or discussions about finances and purchases. They may spend more late nights at work, or pour themselves into a hobby or new area of learning that excludes the partner.

Is it any wonder the sex is not as good?

Consider that every choice you make about how to interact with your partner—whether it's what you say or don't say, what you do or don't do—builds greater intimacy or distance. It's the small moments that create the texture and quality of a relationship.

If you're guilty of taking each other for granted, think back to the thoughtful things you did when the relationship was new. Then do them again, whether it's bringing flowers or taking the time to bake your partner's favorites treats.

Tip: *Content of communication is as vital as technique. If you hope to enjoy consistently good conversation with your partner, you need to open up your conversation beyond everyday practicalities, such as finances and chores. Ask your partner about his or her dreams, or sources of inspiration. Share things you find funny. Delve deep. Look for those subjects that make your partner's eyes light up. Even in a packed life, there should always be time for soulful conversation.*

And never ever use what is revealed in these discussions as ammunition in a subsequent argument. If you do, your partner is likely to clam up and may never become that vulnerable with you again.

Passion Stopper #7: Returning Tit for Tat

It can take a lot of discipline not to lash out at someone who has caused you hurt. Sometimes, you don't even realize that you're harboring hurt or anger, and then, all of a sudden, you find yourself saying something you never intended to say. As the words come out of your mouth, the feelings behind them are a surprise to you, too.

Real intimacy can only take place when both partners feel safe enough to "let down" and be truly vulnerable. Mutual sniping prevents both of you from letting down your guard enough to reach a satisfying level of intimacy.

How do you stop a "slip-up" like this from escalating?

Apologize if you can. Tell your partner you had no idea you were harboring anger or negative feelings. Set aside some time to talk when you can have a relaxed—rather than hurried—conversation. Then promise yourself to be more attentive to your own feelings, catching hurt or anger before it has a chance to go "underground." The next time you notice that something hurts, angers or offends you, explore why you feel that way. When you understand why something upset you, you have a better chance of explaining it to your partner without making him or her feel attacked.

When you do speak, try to go easy on your partner. No one is perfect, and neither are human relationships. Realize this, so you don't set impossible standards for your partner.

If you notice your partner is feeling aggrieved, ask if there is something you should talk about. In either case, strive for a friendly—rather than blaming—exploration of what happened and why it was so hurtful. Genuinely try to see things from your partner's point of view. Try to come to a resolution that works for both of you. This will go much further toward fostering your goal of a mutually satisfying intimate relationship than the temporary "thrill" of winning an argument.

If you are the one accused of being hurtful, a simple "I'm very sorry I hurt you. I didn't mean to" may be more effective than any explanation or justification. These may make your partner feel that you don't take his or her feelings seriously, and fear that you might not be any more considerate in the future. If you typically try to explain yourself, see what happens when you just say, "I'm sorry." You'll be astonished at the power of those words.

Passion-Stopper #8: Hiding, Rather Than Telling the Truth

Honesty isn't just the best policy between lovers; it's the only policy. If you're truly interested in an intimate relationship, you'll want your lover to see you for what you truly are. And if you aren't, don't worry—he or she will eventually see you for what you truly are, as well as for being an insincere person.

Being honest may sometimes make you feel vulnerable. Good. Lovers need to open up and feel vulnerable around one another to establish trust and intimacy. This is absolutely vital to sustained good sex.

Even if you don't tell the truth, nonverbal cues may betray you. If your lover tells you that he or she is willing to listen to your ideas, but does so with a scowl and arms crossed, it's obvious that he or she isn't telling the whole truth. If you want your partner to trust you, make sure that the messages you send through body language are congruent with the words you say. If you're feeling angry, say so. Don't say "I'm not angry" with a clenched jaw, or "I'm fine" in a tight, clipped tone that makes it clear that you are not. Own up to what you feel. If you want to say, "I wish I weren't so angry but that's how I feel right now," that's honest, too. Remember, intimacy isn't limited to sharing the "nice" parts of you, but all of you, in ways that honor your partner as much as yourself.

Keeping quiet on important matters to keep the peace, or hiding activities you suspect your partner won't like, will only backfire.

Everything that is pushed down, or done on the sly, has a way of surfacing. Consider, too, that the energy spent keeping that "unacceptable" part of you hidden is energy that's unavailable for pleasure.

While we're on the subject of honesty, women, never fake an orgasm. It can interfere with trust in your relationship and prevent you from exploring new and more satisfying ways to bring sexual fulfillment.

Tip: *Agree to resolve all differences before climbing into bed. It will help you get a better night's sleep and insure that you'll never wake up angry with one another in the morning. Complete your discussion with a real hug. By wrapping your arms around one another and pressing against each other's chests, you'll break down barriers and replace them with "welcome" mats.*

Establishing the Foundation for Extra-ordinary Sex Together

Eliminating the passion-stoppers in your relationship will do more than just eliminate tension. It may also unleash desire that was blocked before. If you are wise, you will let this unleashed desire carry the two of you forward on a journey of sexual discovery.

To keep yourselves moving forward, make the commitment to "go for it" in your relationship. Make a decision right now to set aside time regularly to explore the ideas, techniques and exercises in this book.

Also commit to establishing a solid foundation from which your sexual life can take off. The following set of principals, as outlined by

Dr. Sandra R. Scantling and Sue Browder in the book, *Ordinary Women, Extraordinary Sex*, as well as in our video series, "Dr. Sandra Scantling's Ordinary Couples, Extraordinary Sex" video, will help solidify that foundation:

1. Assert your needs and respect your partner's boundaries. Let your partner know if anything is unpleasant or uncomfortable for you.
2. Put away old hurts and angers. Don't let yesterday's disagreements or resentments become today's reality.
3. Focus on pleasure, not measure. Remember that sex is not an Olympic event that we rate on a scale from one to ten. It's not about keeping score or counting orgasms. Rather it's about being in the here and now and enjoying the sensations of the moment.
4. Break old patterns. Find new ways to make your loving exciting and fresh. Don't use the same routines and fall into a sexual rut. Creativity is the best antidote to boredom.
5. Treat each other like company. Don't treat strangers better than your lover. Your partner is probably the most important person in your life and deserves to be treated that way.
6. Make time for each other. Spontaneity is best, but scheduled time is fine. Your relationship must take a key position on your priority list if it's to flourish.
7. Communicate clearly. Listen to your partner and make sure you really understood what's being said. This will take a little practice, but don't be discouraged. You'll be surprised at how easily this can be learned.

8. Learn to concentrate on all of your senses. All pleasure is experienced through the senses. Each time you are with your partner, you have an opportunity to practice ways to rediscover sensual enjoyments.

Why It's Important to Have Those Conversations About Sex

When you're feeling disappointed sexually, it may seem easier to talk about everything else but that. You're not alone. Studies conducted by leading universities across the country consistently report that sex is one of the most difficult topics for partners to talk about with each other. One survey found that only 41 percent of women have ever discussed their sex life with their partners, or told them what turns them on. That's sad.

People who don't talk with their partners about what they like—and don't like—when they are making love are not going to achieve the same level of satisfaction as couples who do. Lowered levels of satisfaction can lead to resentment, which will dampen desire, creating a tailspin in the relationship. If you don't talk with each other, minor differences can swell into a major crisis.

Reluctance to talk about sex with your partner is usually rooted in some kind of insecurity. Maybe you think your partner will feel that you're selfish if you assert your needs, or that you're too forward. Maybe you're nervous that your comments will make your partner feel inadequate. That doesn't have to be the case. It's all in the way you say it. Here are suggestions for making your talk productive and intimacy enhancing:

• Affirm your love, before you bring up anything difficult. Let the partner know that the objectionable behavior or comment is interfering with your ability to express that love.

• Focus on the good. Compliment your lover on his or her appearance, personal qualities and bedroom skills. Encouraging words foster endearing feelings and enchanting sex.

• Frame your desire as a request for something new, rather than a criticism of what isn't being done right.

• Don't pass judgment. An expression of disapproval can shut down sexual communication lines for a long time. Don't criticize your partner's ideas about sex, even if you find them unpleasant. Instead, ask for further explanation. Also, avoid critiques of your lover's sexual performance, as they inevitably lead to resentment. Offer encouragement and suggestions instead.

• Make a game of it. A good way to alleviate the tension of discussing sex is to put it in the context of a simple game. That's how many adolescents get over the awkwardness of the subject. There's no reason you can't find success with that tactic as an adult.

• Ask for requests. Let your lover know you're open to suggestions.

• Talk before sex. Letting your partner know exactly what you like in bed and how you like it is informative, intimate and arousing.

• Talk during sex. Obviously, you don't want to keep up a running patter that interferes with your ability to revel in the physical sensations, but do tell your partner when something feels great, ask for a different kind of stimulation if you need it, or ask your partner what he or she would enjoy next. Moans and screams of delight don't hurt either.

• Talk after sex. A simple "thank you" followed by intense cuddling can do the trick. You can talk about anything really. Just make sure to keep open the lines of communication once the sex is over.

• If you can't bring yourself to assert what you want in bed (or elsewhere), find a competent counselor who can help you build your confidence. You might find it easier to talk through fears or worries with a "neutral," well-trained counselor than take the risk of complete disclosure in your intimate relationship. That will come later, as your sense of self builds.

IMPROVING YOUR LISTENING SKILLS

Sometimes, insecurities or other fears can get in the way of truly hearing your partner. And that can set the stage for a whopper of a fight, because no one likes being disregarded after making the effort to explain what they want or don't want. To prevent the ill will that's bound to follow:

• Listen deeply. Bring all of your attention to what your partner is saying. And if you have too much on your mind to be able to bring all of yourself to the conversation, be honest enough to say so. Commit to a time when you can be available.

• Don't interrupt until your partner is finished. Agree that you will do this for each other. Sometimes, simply being heard can change the way your partner feels. It can dissolve tension and reopen the heart. Listening without interruption can help you learn more about each other.

• Strike the right balance between listening and revealing your own feelings. Don't allow yourselves to fall into a rut where one partner is doing all the talking and the other is doing all the listening. If one partner seems less talkative, the more talkative one can ask questions and draw the other out. Some people are naturally more gifted at expressing themselves than their partners. It's important that the more skilled partner help the other to become equally skilled, so that conversations become a mutual sharing rather than one-upmanship.

As Michelle learned, what's important "is listening with an open heart. It's not just being able to hear what my husband says, and repeat it. There's more to it than that. I think it's really listening with an openness and an acceptance. I think more than anything else, we want to be accepted by our life partner."

Establishing good communication, heeding the principles above, and experimenting with the techniques and exercises that follow will help you go beyond self-imposed sexual limits, explore new vistas of sexuality and learn how to get the most out of sexual pleasure. Being honest about what you expect from sex and sharing your fantasies can open up whole new dimensions of pleasure—dimensions that may even take you beyond your fondest hopes for your sexual relationship.

WAYS TO DRAW CLOSER

To keep things heated up between the two of you, establish a few love and intimacy rituals. Choose ones that feel great to both of you. These ideas may inspire you:

- *Mark each departure and reunion with a genuine expression of love. Hug, kiss, or whisper something sweet. This makes it clear that you consider your time together a sweet gift, and that you value the connection.*

- *Turn cuddling into a daily ritual. Spend as much time as you can hugging, spooning, smooching, stroking and smiling at one another before you go to sleep each night—and before you get out of bed each morning. And when you can spare a few minutes at any other point during the day.*

- *Share a hobby. Find an activity besides sex you can both enjoy and do regularly together.*

- *Play games. A little friendly competition gets the juices flowing and helps you get to know your partner better.*

• Share a new adventure each month. Pick something you've never done before. Go sailing, rollerblading or attend a salsa night at a local club. Seek the new together so that you continue to grow and learn together.

• Walk and talk. A 20-minute walk after dinner not only burns off calories, it offers a great forum for conversation and mini-adventures. Exercising together in just about any way can be a good, regular bonding experience.

• Share as many meals as possible with your partner. Do whatever it takes—get up a half-hour earlier to have breakfast together before work, schedule a lunch date, get a babysitter and go out to dinner. Eating together deepens bonds of intimacy. Establish at least one meal a day as sacred time together.

• Surprise your beloved with little gifts. Birthday, holiday and anniversary presents are nice, if not required. But an unexpected little something every now and then is extra nice. The gift doesn't have to be expensive or elaborate. It should just show that you're thinking of him or her.

• Show your partner extra consideration. Some people feel so secure in their relationships they put much more effort into pleasing others. But this doesn't serve your goal of building a mutually fulfilling relationship, and may create resentment. If you haven't done so, move your beloved to the top of your "special

favors" list. Partners deserve and require special treatment more than clients, bosses, or parents. Your kids are the only ones in the same league. By showing your partner he or she comes "first" with you, you build the kind of good will that will return to you tenfold. This sets the relationship on a strong, positive course, so that good becomes great, and great becomes "Wow. This relationship is the best thing that ever happened to me. I wouldn't trade my partner for the world."

About the Sinclair Videos

The 10 Secrets to Great Sex, designed as a companion to the Sinclair Video library, is complete unto itself. It contains much of the same information you will find in the company's video library, including The Better Sex Video Series®. If you would like to see a video presentation of the sexual techniques desribed in this book, you do have the option of watching the videos. We list the relevant videos at the end of each chapter.

You can order them through Bettersex.com, the web store of the Sinclair Intimacy Institute, or call 1-800-955-0888. You will also find top-of-the-line sex toys. The Better Sex Video Series®, and our entire line of over 50 instructional videos, were created in concert with leading sexuality educators, family and marriage counselors, and therapists to provide the latest sexual health education.

For videos that relate specifically to Secret #1, "Make the Decision to Go for It," see *Dr. Sandra Scantling's Ordinary Couples, Extraordinary Sex,* Video Series Volumes 1-3: *Discovering Extraordinary Sex, Getting Creative with Sex,* and *Keeping Sex Extraordinary.*

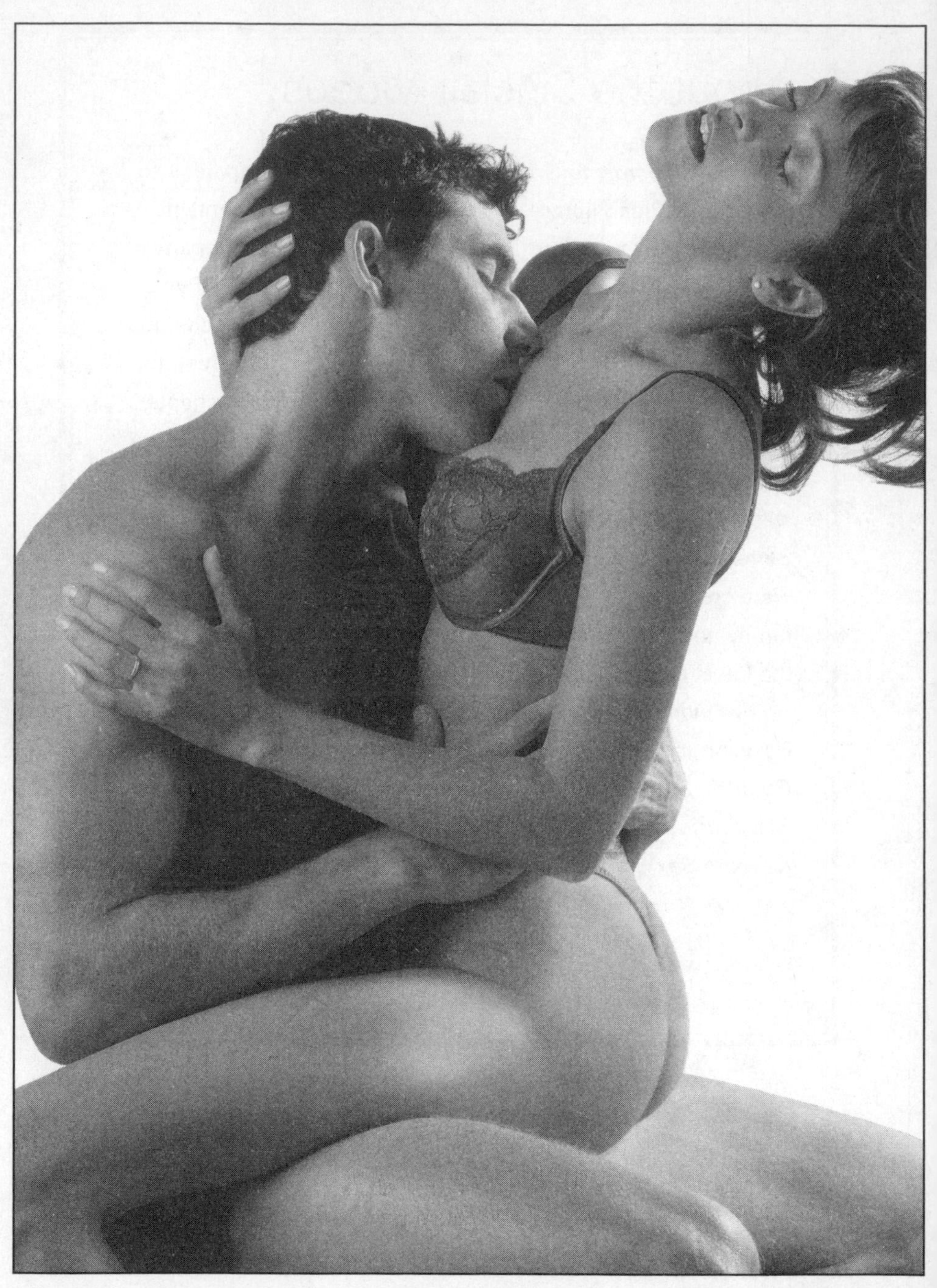

SECRET #2

Focus on Whole-Body Pleasure

> *To lovers, touch is metamorphosis. All the parts of their bodies seem to change, and seem to become something different and better.*
>
> —JOHN CHEEVER

Dawn wasn't climbing the corporate ladder. She was headed up the express elevator. She organized each day around her career, establishing and achieving new goals while advancing toward her long-term goal of becoming her company's CEO. Dawn applied this same approach to sex with her fiancé Brad, another corporate go-getter. Each knew exactly what he or she wanted in bed, and how to achieve it. They understood how to quickly stimulate and achieve orgasm in themselves and in one another.

While Brad and Dawn found this focus exciting at first, they soon felt themselves drifting emotionally and then physically from one another. They talked about the problem, but concluded that as long as they scheduled in enough "quality sex time" and kept the orgasms coming, everything would work out. But as time went on, they found that their intimacy faded and resentment toward one another increased. The relationship began to sour. They each began to see it as a hindrance to the achievement of their other life goals, rather than as a source of emotional and physical support that enhanced their life.

Goal-oriented thinking may get you a long way in the boardroom. But it's a detour from intimacy and real satisfaction in the bedroom. Focusing on orgasm or other "goals" during sex can make you tense and push you out of the moment, alienating you from the experience, your lover and even your own body. A great, sustained sexual relationship requires a different approach, one that embraces the whole body.

While intercourse and orgasm may seem like the goal of sex, couples who enjoy extraordinary sex know that the real secret is learning to become sensual with each other. That means opening up to whole-body (rather than just genitally-focused) pleasure, and enjoying all of life's delights. They savor the smell of flavored coffee together in the morning, the love communicated through a quick squeeze of the hand when they're out walking together, the sound of their partner's voice on the phone.

They also learn to keep themselves turned on, by surrounding themselves with things that delight their senses. For some individuals, that means indulging in a nice all-body moisturizer after a shower, or keeping fresh flowers in the house. For others, it means amassing a collection of wonderful music and making the time to appreciate it.

This is the secret of people who radiate sex appeal and satisfaction. A supermodel's face or Olympian physique isn't required here. Finding ways to stay turned on—and help your partner stay turned on—are. And that means attuning your mind to pleasure and paying attention, so you don't miss even one exquisite pleasure message your body is trying to send you.

Question: I'd like to try something new, how do I approach my partner?

Variety is the spice of a great sex life. And the possibilities are endless—new games, toys, positions and fantasies are just a few ways to intensify sexual enjoyment in monogamous relationships. And new things can have a snowball effect— as one partner instigates new pleasures, the other partner then wants to reciprocate with imaginative activities. Pretty soon you're having more fun than you ever dreamed possible.

You may be concerned that your partner might experience some resistance to your sexy new idea. This is actually a good sign— it means that you're sensitive to his or her feelings.

Start by talking about what you'd like to try. In all likelihood, your partner will be just as excited as you are. If they do have reservations, work gently through them. It's worth pursuing because growing beyond old sexual boundaries can be a huge turn-on for both partners. Watching a sexual instructional video together is a great way to break the ice and spark communication and ideas. Any discomfort you may feel at first quickly gives way to interest and a quickening of the imagination. Check out the Sinclair Video Library at www.bettersex.com.

THE MIND

Great sex starts in the mind. This is where you choose whether to be attuned to the pleasure of the moment, or to ignore the moment, engaging instead in replaying hurtful experiences from the past, or letting little insecurities become full-blown performance anxiety, or thinking about what comes next, instead of feeling what's happening now. Why let your mind blow your opportunity for really mind-blowing sex? Decide now that you are the one in control. Resolve to practice letting go of self-defeating thinking patterns and focusing on the pleasures of the moment.

Taking the time to relax regularly will help reconnect your mind and body. It lets you stop thinking about where you're headed and start concentrating on where you are, putting you in tune with your body, your mind and your lover.

Start learning to live again in the present tense with this simple exercise: Go to bed a half-hour earlier and wake up a half-hour earlier. If you can't possibly accomplish this on a workday, try it on your next day off. After getting out of bed, choose a quiet room where you can lie down and get comfortable. Close your eyes. Let your stomach rise and fall naturally as you inhale and exhale. This is called belly breathing. Babies breathe this way naturally. As people grow up, they learn to suck in their stomachs. This interferes with the way the body wants to breathe.

Use this belly breathing exercise for sensual relaxation. As you inhale and exhale, focus on the sound of your breath and let your thoughts quiet down. Try to think of nothing at all. But if you get some stray sexy insights, just let them drift peacefully through your mind. On the other hand, if you find yourself thinking about your job or your grocery list, move on to this more advanced exercise:

Relaxation Exercise

Start with the tips of your toes. Tense them up and then release them. Enjoy the sensation of relief in your feet. And then travel up your body—tensing and releasing your calves, thighs, groin, hands etc., and enjoying the sensations until you reach the top of your head. Then, finally, just let yourself drift and feel quiet. Let your mind and body become one again.

You can use this exercise throughout the day—sitting at your desk, before lunch, on the way home from work. If you don't think you have time, think again. Relaxing and reconnecting with yourself actually energizes your body and clears your mind. Consider it a small investment that will bring great returns in increased efficiency. Relaxation will also pay big dividends in your sex life. In this relaxed state, you'll start to feel in tune with what your body wants and needs, instead of constantly trying to goad it toward present goals. You'll find moving toward your sexual needs and desires becomes instinctive. Take this mind set into the bedroom next time you make love. Rather than focusing on achieving orgasm—thinking about it so intently that you push it away—just exist in the moment. Feel your breath, your lover's touch, the sensations on your skin and those within. Accept the pleasures that your body gives you. Don't compare them with yesterday's joys, or regard them as a bridge to cross to reach climax. Great sex honors each and every feeling and moment.

The Body

One Saturday after an early morning yoga class, Dawn returned to bed where Brad still lay asleep. She continued a deep breathing exercise from the class as she lay next to her lover, becoming more and more at ease and tuned into her mind and body. Then something delightful happened. As he began waking up, Brad stirred and accidentally tickled Dawn with the sheets. The soft edge of the sheets against her leg felt wonderful. She returned the favor. Then she leaned over and stroked his shoulders. Brad smiled and Dawn rubbed his arm. He reached over and stroked her legs. Now they were both smiling.

For the next ten minutes, they took turns tickling and stroking one another. This little game actually opened up a door that had remained closed since early in their relationship.

For the first time in a long time, they were enjoying the most basic sensory pleasures of being together. Instead of working toward a sexual goal, they were spontaneously playing for the sheer sensual delight of it. And in doing so, they were connecting at a deeper level than they ever had before.

Arousing the Senses

Engaging all of your senses—touch, sight, sound, smell and taste—in sex play makes it a multidimensional experience. Each sense has much to contribute. If the stress of modern living has dulled your senses, you can revitalize them by lovingly exploring each one on your own, then experimenting with ways you can make exploration of that sense a delight for you and your partner.

Touch, the sense most connected with sexual pleasure, is the language of love. Loving strokes, relaxing rubs and teasing tickles offer a delicious way for lovers to express their needs and affection. Too often, however, we reserve the pleasure of touch for the bedroom. While it certainly belongs there, it also plays an important part in every aspect of life. Glory in the things you touch every day —the warm water coming out of your bathroom faucet in the morning, the soft soap you spread over your body, the rug beneath your bare feet, the softness of your own skin. Then venture further. Stop to touch the roses in your garden, running your fingers over their silky petals. Move your hands over a smooth vase. Brush a feather against your cheeks, arms, stomach and thighs. Enjoy the textures, as well as the sensations they stir in you.

Practice using touch to reconnect with your lover outside the bedroom. Next time you're sitting together, reach over and gently stroke his or her hair, neck and arms. Hold hands when you walk. Rub your foot up and down his or her leg beneath the dinner table. Give each other massages, using your hands to communicate your affection and to receive his or her messages about what movements feel best.

Great lovers are great touchers. So stay in touch with yours wherever and however you can.

GETTING IN TOUCH WITH TOUCH

Touch remains the one sense essential to lovemaking. You could make love without seeing, hearing, tasting or smelling. But it is impossible without some form of touch. To experience the primacy of touch, try this game with your lover:

Dim the lights in your bedroom and play a CD featuring low-key ambient music—something that will cover up other sounds while not drawing attention to itself. Make sure the room temperature will comfortably accommodate a naked body. Then take off your clothes, get onto the bed and simultaneously tie blindfolds onto each other.

Begin touching. Start with light grazes and slow strokes. Move to longer strokes that cover your lover's entire body. Though the occasional sigh or giggle will slip out, try to stay as silent as possible. Deprived of your vision and with your other senses operating at a minimum, your sense of touch will be intensified—on both the giving and receiving ends. Continue stroking one another's bodies. Explore places you may have never touched before—between your lover's toes, behind his or her knees, the top of the ears, the back of the neck. You will find erotic zones you may not have known existed. Proceed at a deliberate pace, staying away from the genitals, nipples or other erogenous zones. Let your hands glide their way to new places and movements. If you continue with this long enough, your sense of touch will reach new heights. You'll feel deeply connected to your body and to your lover's body. Resist the urge to rip off your blindfolds and engage in conventional sex until you can't take it anymore. Or simply end with a full embrace and lay in one another's arms.

The Art of Touch

Massage may well be the ultimate form of nonverbal communication. Regular massage sessions help lovers convey affection, revitalize one another and learn more about the other's erogenous zones. Some couples enjoy it as much as sex.

You don't need to be an expert masseuse to give your lover a wonderful erotic massage. The most important element of a successful massage is being present with your partner, giving generously and attuning yourself to your beloved's body.

Prepare for the massage by choosing a good oil. A scented oil can evoke a sensual mood. An unscented oil may be a wise choice for lovers with sensitive skin. Most bath & body and health food shops carry a variety of massage oils. Sinclair has its own brand, Better Sex Massage Oil. Try one with lavender or chamomile if you want to induce relaxation, or peppermint if you want to stimulate the body. You can also blend your own, using a mild vegetable oil and a scented flower or plant oil. This will cost less than premixed varieties, and gives you more creative freedom.

Once you have the oil, heat it to a comfortable temperature before applying it to your partner. If you can't do that, at least warm the oil up on your hands before it touches your partner's body. You also want to set the thermostat a little higher than normal (around 75 degrees). Or light the fireplace if you're lucky enough to have one. And gather some clean sheets, pillows and blankets to keep your partner cozy. If your partner has back problems, keep an extra folded blanket on hand to place under his or her knees and take pressure off the lower back.

continued . . .

. . . Continued

Pick out some soft music that will relax your partner and help you get into a massage rhythm. Then dim the lights, or burn some candles in the room. When you are ready to start, rub your palms together to get the energy flowing in your hands.

Of course, you can use more than your hands during the massage. Use your lips to massage your partner's temples. Flutter your eyelashes over your partner's cheekbones. Blow on your partner's nipples. Sweep your hair down the length of your lover's back.

Stroke softly at first, especially if you're massaging a delicate area like the abdomen or neck. Using a light touch will allow you to massage longer, and build erotic anticipation rather than tiring you and your partner. You can always deepen your strokes at your partner's request.

As you massage, attend to every part of the body, including the backs of the knees, the hands and feet, the head, the lips, the eyes. See what delights your partner the most. Finally, think of a gift with no strings attached, rather than a trade. Certainly, in the overall relationship, you should strike for balance between giving and receiving. But this doesn't mean that you should each give and receive a massage in the same session. Allow the partner who's on the receiving end the option of fully relaxing and focusing on his or her pleasure. Don't worry, you'll receive plenty in return.

While touch can be very arousing, information received through the eyes can also bring instant arousal. Some individuals are intensely visual. If your partner is, take extra care to appeal to their sense of aesthetics with your grooming, choice of dress and artful arrangement of the area where you make love. Create a visual feast, choosing those items you know will appeal to your lover. If your lover doesn't get the hint, suggest what he or she can do to return the favor to you.

Sound also wields power as a sexual enhancer—or downer. The whine of a neighbor's leaf blower can undermine an erotic setting as easily as the throbbing bass on a soulful CD gets your mojo humming. As you become more at ease with your body and lover, annoying sounds should prove less distracting (you may even stop noticing them altogether). In the meantime, experiment with different sounds and musical selections when setting up a romantic environment.

Start with the obvious choices—a crackling fire, your favorite romantic music, a miniature waterfall fountain. Then try some sounds that might not seem sexy at first. Making love to a loud, frenetic jazz CD or the rumble of a clothes dryer can provide an interesting and exciting sonic alternative.

Still, the human voice remains the most powerfully sexual sound. Whisper sweet nothings into your lover's ear. Compliment him or her on appearance, smell and taste. Express your feelings—affection, excitement, commitment. Say you can't wait to get romantic. Don't wait until you're in bed, lean over anywhere—at a restaurant, during an opera, on an escalator—and let your feelings and intentions be known.

Next, you might want to express things that aren't so sweet at a few decibels above a whisper. Many people enjoy sexy talk during lovemaking. The important thing is to carefully gauge your lover's preferences. Discuss the subject after sex. You may be surprised and excited at what your partner has to say, and wants to hear.

Nonverbal expression can be even more powerful. Regard the sounds your lover makes during sex as a wonderful music. While grunts, moans and sighs may not necessarily fall into your definition of music, remember: these are the melodies of arousal, excitement, pleasure and satisfaction. (If you're not convinced, check out Sinclair's "Advanced Sexual Fantasy" video for a hot scene between some prehistorically attired lovers who communicate with primal urgency.)

Lastly, remember the most important sound lovers can share: conversation. Reserve romantic settings for discussing subjects you don't get around to in normal situations. Talk about art, the music you're listening to, your deepest desires and secret dreams. You may find whole new levels of intimacy and appreciation opening up, along with some interesting sexual adventures.

The sense of smell is one of the most evocative senses and one of the most mysterious. A whiff of perfume can take you back decades and open the door to vivid memories. Despite its subtlety, smell has a powerful impact on human sexuality. In fact, the olfactory sense is processed by the same part of the brain—the deep limbic system, which is responsible for our feelings of connection to others.

To awaken your sense of smell, try these tips. Savor the smell of your coffee in the morning. Air out your car and spruce it up with a little incense. Decorate your office with plants that will filter out pollutants and replace them with clean, natural odors. Pay particular attention to the aromatic environment of your bedroom. Scented candles, perfumes and colognes, flowers, and beautiful smelling soaps will make a nice impression on your lover.

If you and your partner would like to create a gourmet menu for your noses, try this fun exercise. Go out and collect a variety of wonderful-smelling items (perfume and bath shops, grocery stores, flower shops and even clothing and hardware stores can be a source of erotic smells). Then, when you get home, take turns closing your eyes and trying to identify each item just by smell. Gauge the effect each smell has on your moods and memories. Make a list of favorites, then use these scents to enhance future romantic experiences.

Some people believe that great food is better than sex. But why choose one when you can have both? Food and sex are two of life's most nourishing sensual pleasures.

You and your lover can turn even ordinary meals into romantic rituals. Whether dining on Chinese takeout or a home-cooked feast, you can treat every meal like the celebration of life that it is. Forget about your worries and your cares. Light some candles or dim the lights, put on some soft music, and relax and enjoy each other's company.

Take the time to really taste your food. Savor your meal with all your senses, not just the taste buds. Appreciate the colors, the textures, and the aromas. Tempt your palate with new flavors and new combinations. And tempt each other with charming conversation and flirtatious looks. This works as well at a weekday breakfast as a Friday night dinner.

It can work wonderfully in the bedroom as well. Delight in breaking that unwritten rule of "no eating in bed." Share dessert in the bed. Share spoonfuls of ice cream or cake, then exchange kisses. Feed each other strawberries. Use a honey bear to drizzle sweetness onto your partner's tongue. Make your lover's tummy into a sexy treat with whipped cream and a maraschino cherry. It's one of those rare occasions when you can have your cake, and eat it too. While you're there, experiment and see how many different "tastes" you can find on your lover's bare body.

Bon Appètite

Stimulate your senses regularly to keep your sensory awareness in peak form. Think of it as exercising your sensory muscles. Games offer a great way to consistently engage the mind and open the senses to pleasure. If you'd like to have some fun with your partner and expand your sensual repertoire at the same time, try relationship board games such as "More Foreplay." A sexual "spin the bottle" for grown-ups, the game helps you select body parts for special attention, and tells you how long—as well as how—to stimulate them. The game allows for a seemingly infinite variety of sensual experiences—from mild to wild, from titillating to mind-boggling. It may take you at least a year or two to work through all of the possibilities of that game.

If you'd like to see a visual presentation of the material in this chapter, refer to the following videos from the Sinclair Intimacy Institute Video Library: *Dr. Sandra Scantling's Discovering Unforgettable Sex* Volume 1: *Five Steps to Unforgettable Sex,* and *The Joy of Erotic Massage.* Also consider the CD *"Aphrodisia,"* which contains a selection of erotic music.

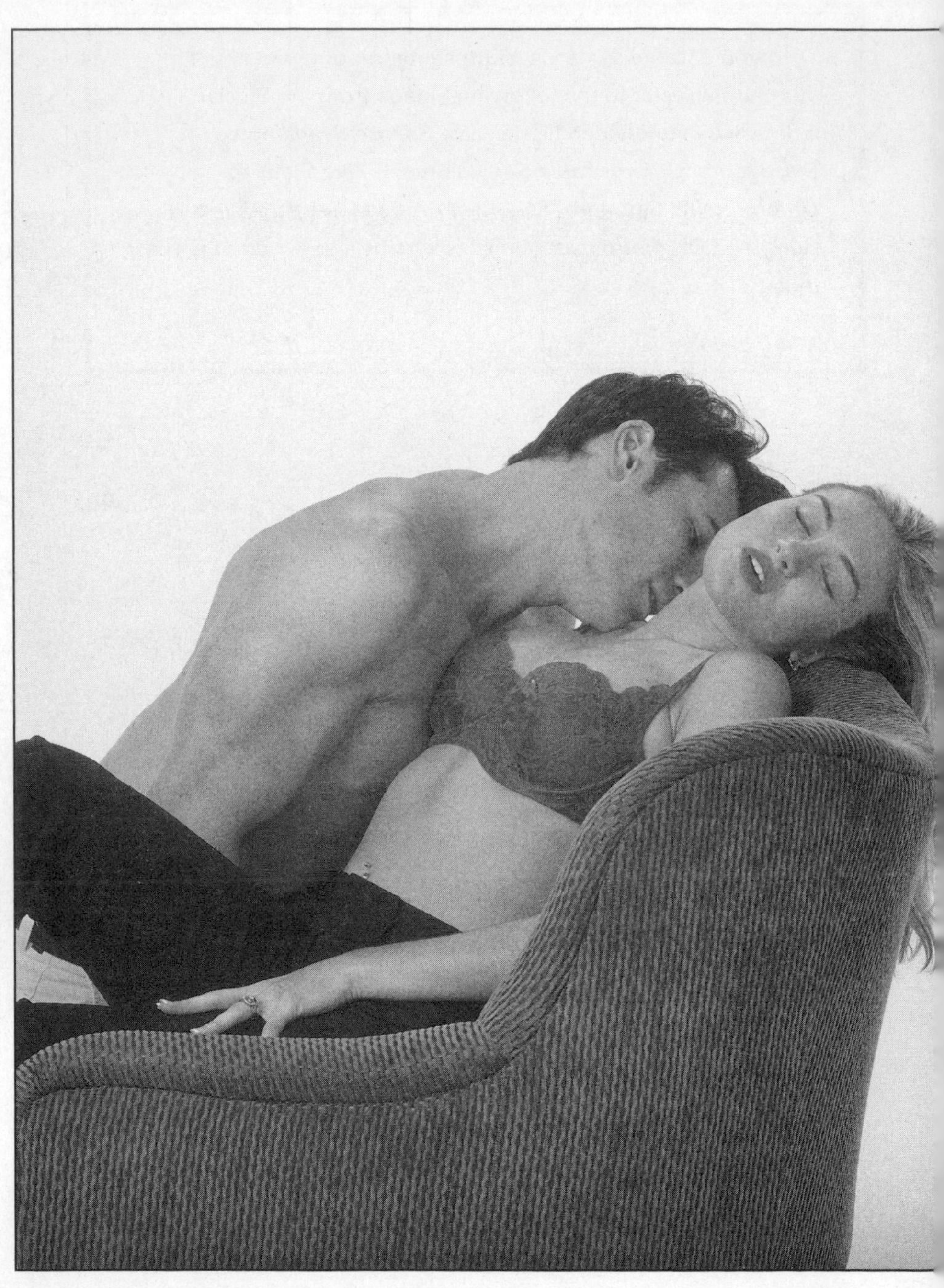

SECRET #3

Approach Seduction as an Art Form

> It is not enough to conquer; one must know how to seduce.
>
> —VOLTAIRE

Lauren and Thomas worked long hours at their respective offices, then came home to carc for their three young children. They never seemed to find enough alone time for sex, let alone the energy to seduce each other. Each continued to entertain erotic thoughts and feel sexual longing, but they rechanneled the passion into private fantasies, rather than back into the relationship. That only drove them further apart. After awhile, they began feeling less like a loving couple than platonic coworkers on a long-term project.

If this is happening in your relationship, don't wait any longer to turn things around. Great lovers make time for intimacy. And they know how to turn their partners on so resistance dissolves. In fact, the greatest lovers are great seducers—they enjoy the chase and lure as much as the capture. They are always inventing new ways to make this next seduction even more fun and exciting than the last. They understand that keeping things "hot" year after year requires striking the right balance between variety and familiarity. Instead of sticking to the "tried and true," they look for new ways to surprise and tantalize their beloved.

If you are in a long-term relationship, realize that the art of seduction is even more essential for you than for single folks. Don't ever think that a relationship has "matured" beyond the stage where you no longer need to sexually entice one another. That attitude will create boredom—and perhaps even resentment—between you. Men, this is an especially important point for you to commit to memory. Even though your idea of a great evening is a night of great sex, surveys show that women would rather watch a movie. So if you want her to want what you want, you have to help her along a little. If you know her well, you can probably figure out what to do to completely take her mind off that foreign film she's been dying to see.

Let Anticipation Build

The lover who treats seduction almost as an afterthought, timing it just before anticipated lovemaking, may not get as generous a response as the lover who knows how to let anticipation build through the days, or week. The first can make the intended feel manipulated; the second, cared for. So go ahead and express your lusty feelings as you cuddle, do yard work together, debate politics or share a midnight walk with your mate. Desire for physical union often arises during these "everyday" moments. This is especially important if your lives are packed full and there hardly seems time to cultivate romance, given responsibilities at work and home.

Fortunately, seduction doesn't have to be time consuming. A staged, grand gesture can be nice. But a series of quick, subtle gestures throughout the day can generate sexual attraction just as effectively. Perhaps that involves bringing your partner coffee in bed in the morning, or calling midday from work to say, "I can't wait to see you. I want you." Or maybe it's that call that says, "I know how hard you've been working. How about if I bring dinner home?" Or "I've cooked up a little surprise for you. What time did you say you were getting off from work?" This is how you forge the connections that will ramp up the energy for your next intimate encounter.

Finding Opportunities for Seduction Throughout the Day

Great lovers understand that seduction doesn't necessarily lead quickly to sex. Some of the most delicious seductions take place over a relatively lengthy period of time. You may not have the time or energy to have sex every day. But you and your partner can seduce one another throughout the day.

If you'd like to end up back in bed for sex with your partner at some point during the day, start setting the stage when you wake up in the morning. Stroking your lover's hair or cuddling up close first thing in the morning sets a tone for the day's interactions. (As always, be respectful of each other's moods and preferences. If your partner isn't a "morning person" give him or her time to ease into the day.)

How Some Lovers Create an Atmosphere of Seduction

When he arrived home after a long day at work, Tim sensed something was different. He saw that his wife, Lauren, had attached a note to their front door. He was expecting it to say that she'd gone out to shop or that the oven was broken. Instead, it read, "Come inside, my lover, and follow your path to pleasure."

Suddenly energized and excited, Tim did as he was told. Inside, he found a red string leading to the kitchen. The string was attached to the handle of an ice bucket with a bottle of champagne inside. A second note there instructed him to go to the living room and hit the "Play" button on the cassette player. When he did, Lauren's voice came over the stereo speakers telling him to head to the bathroom with the champagne. Sexy, jazzy music followed.

His excitement building, Tim entered the bathroom. He found Lauren sitting in a bubble bath surrounded by candlelight, holding two champagne glasses. She beckoned him into the tub. There they drank champagne and took turns soaping and rinsing one another. Afterwards, Lauren wrapped Tim a large soft towel and led him into the bedroom. She'd replaced the regular light bulb with one that emitted a soft red glow throughout the room. They laid down together on the bed, now covered in new satin sheets, and enjoyed the best sex they'd had in years.

Games like these are very effective at arousing your lover. But you don't have to go to as much effort as Tim and Lauren. Try filling a vase with slips of paper naming individual body parts and another vase with a list of sensations, then taking turns picking one slip from each vase. Or play "Lover's Request," a game in which answering a question correctly allows you to name your price. (If you give the wrong answer, your lover chooses.) You and your lover can create the questions as you go. You can also stage a treasure hunt, with you and your lover searching for different items (brushes, lotions, etc.) hidden around the house. The winner gets to say how the item will be used in foreplay. Playing at games like these helps you add fun to your time together. There's no reason why seduction has to be serious business. Lightening it up can help you relax and enjoy each other more.

If you shower together, use the opportunity to lather, stroke and rinse your partner (especially with a removable showerhead.) Then help your lover to towel off afterwards. Pause a minute to run your fingers along a "sweet spot" you've discovered during massage. Send your lover suggestive looks as you dress.

If it's a workday, consider tucking a romantic card or note into a purse or briefcase. Does your lover have to endure a long commute? Make a tape for the car stereo of you whispering sexy thoughts.

Even if there are chores to do at the end of a long workday, look for ways to express your affection and desire as you complete them. Make grocery shopping an erotic adventure with imaginative talk. Whisper something sexy into your lover's ear at a PTA meeting. ("I know you're bored now, but I have something at home that I think you'll find very exciting.") Get playful doing yard work.

At the end of the day, help each other wind down. Realize that stress overload can undermine sexual desire, and may even affect sexual performance. So hug each other. Exchange neck and shoulder massages. Share words of love and encouragement. Fantasize together about a vacation you'd like to take together. Above all, make each other laugh; humor releases tension and puts things into perspective. The more relaxed you make one another feel, the more likely you'll ease into sex.

If your days are so stressful that you feel too worn out for sex, consider scheduling time to exercise together. Regular exercise will not only raise your energy level, but also bring back that glow of well being, and improve blood flow to vital organs, which will increase your pleasure. If you have the privacy, try naked partner yoga and stretching. Consider new uses for home fitness machines. A weight bench can be used for more than just bench-pressing.

Using Dinner to Stimulate Your "Other" Appetite

If you can manage a dinner for just the two of you, take it to the hilt. Pop a strawberry into your lover's mouth. Feed each other with your fingers. Just avoid overeating and overdrinking (which leads to lethargy). Remember that one or two drinks can put you "in the mood," but more than that can put you out of commission. That's because alcohol is a depressant. Dinner in bed is especially nice. Arrange for "room service" just like you get in fine hotels. Choose "racy" desserts like chocolate mouse over vanilla ice cream. Feed one another chocolate mousse by dipping your fingers into the bowl, then into your lover's mouth. Exchange chocolate kisses. You can take it a delicious step further by spreading the dessert onto different parts of one another's bodies, then licking it off. This definitely qualifies as foreplay.

If your days are too packed even for this, try scheduling time for sex. This may seem a bit forced at first, but once you get over the initial awkwardness, you can develop scheduled sex as an occasion that you'll both look forward to. Write it in your date book. Plan your day around it. Make a flirtatious reminder to call to your mate. Use your organizational skills to make it happen.

Become a Student of Seduction

There's nothing more seductive than confidence. Confidence often comes from knowledge. So if you want to confidently seduce your partner, study him or her. Look for clues about what turns your beloved on. Consider not only what has worked in the past, but also what you can do to meet the needs of the moment.

If you need inspiration, look to the movies and/or music your partner enjoys. Think back over times you ended up having terrific sex together. How did it start? Look for patterns in your partner's responses. Is your lover more easily aroused in the morning, afternoon or evening? Do direct or indirect approaches work best? What specific kinds of clothing, accessories, settings turn your lover on?

Be attentive to detail, or you may miss what's important. That foot rub earlier in the evening may have aroused your partner more than the late-night carriage ride to the hotel. Be careful, however, not to jump to conclusions. Consider your new insights "theories" until you test them out and see how well they work. Look to nonverbal clues for confirmation. A sigh or other physical response that suggests openness to physical intimacy will tell you much more than words ever could have; so will a slight backing off or turning away.

You can also learn a lot just by asking your partner. Begin the conversation by expressing your love and your desire to please your partner. Then ask fun, positive, nonthreatening questions such as, "What can I do that I'm not doing to make it impossible for you to resist me?" or "What could I wear that would raise your temperature?" "What kinds of touch—and where—make you melt?" Break the ice by volunteering some of your special turn-ons. Compliment your lover on the ways he or she has turned you on in the past. Say you'd like to return the favor. Eventually, your partner should open up. As you listen, be as nonjudgmental and accepting as possible. Remember that your goal is greater intimacy. If you express anger or disappointment over what your lover reveals, you've just defeated your purpose. So listen respectfully, with genuine curiosity and unconditional acceptance. This honors your partner, and there is nothing like being honored when speaking your truth. That forges deep and intimate bonds between lovers.

SUREFIRE WAYS TO REPEL YOUR PARTNER

Not all approaches to seduction work every time. But these blunders virtually guarantee failure:

- *Asking for pity. This chases away lust as quickly as body odor.*

- *Smothering your partner. The idea of seduction is to lure your mate to you, not to latch on so he or she can't get away.*

- *Bullying. Nobody likes bullies, much less finds them sexy.*

- *Expecting sex on demand. Your partner is NOT obligated to desire you or fulfill your desire at any given moment. If you expect that, you may wait a long, long time for fulfillment.*

- *Manipulation through guilt. Telling your mate that he or she has done you wrong— and therefore owes you sex—is bound to backfire.*

- *Constant criticism. Talking about how much you disapprove of someone or something isn't going to inspire your listener to approve of you.*

- *Rude behavior. What more needs to be said?*

- *Talking nonstop. This can wear out your lover, which is not the result you intend.*

Using the Element of Surprise to Spice Things Up

The more you get to know your partner, the easier it is to know how to plan surprises that will definitely delight your beloved. A pleasant surprise—whether it's a lusty telegram or a sexy new outfit—sends a charge through the brain and loins. Or the surprise could be a seduction by the partner who usually waits to be seduced. Yep, ladies, this means you. Many men long to be ravished by their women, but always have to take the lead. A man loves it when his partner turns the tables, and makes him feel wanted and needed.

You can also add a little spice by "dressing" for sex. In fact, it can be fun to create a wardrobe around your sexual "moods." Is this a "leather" night, or one that calls for silk and satin? Ladies, a pink lace teddy signals that you're ready for a night of gentle love; while a black corset and high heels suggests something very different. Men, consider whether the occasion calls for silk boxer shorts, or a tush-baring thong. Realize how seductive your outerwear can be. Some women go gaga over guys in tight biking shorts. Others can't resist a man in a well-tailored business suit.

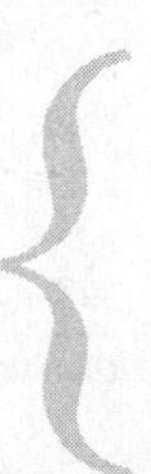

Tip: *Instead of dressing yourself, dress your bed for romance. Surprise your mate with a new bedspread in a sensual color. Scatter rose petals on the pillows. Light candles and place them around the room. Use your imagination to turn your bed into your own personal altar to love.*

Even little things can make a difference. For some couples, for instance, temporary tattoos can be very exciting. Your partner won't be able to resist getting a look at the complete picture of that racy tattoo design peeking out over the top of your pants. A design on a torso or buttock can also provide a tantalizing surprise. Temporary tattoos are now widely available. They're inexpensive and scrub off easily with baby oil or massage oil—rather than soap.

If you don't have much in the way of an intimate wardrobe, take the time to sit down together and talk about what the two of you would like to see the other wear. Negotiate if you have to, but make it fun. Then make your shopping together an adnveture.

At the Border of Seduction and Foreplay

Seduction doesn't end the minute you two are buck-naked together. Great lovers treat seduction as a form of foreplay—and foreplay as an extension of seduction. With some new tricks, you can make foreplay as satisfying as the main event.

Try going longer than usual, for instance. Extending foreplay over the course of an hour, or even a day, builds anticipation and heightens pleasure, response and desire. It can also lead to window-shattering orgasms. Of course, there's nothing wrong with ripping off one another's clothes for the occasional quickie, provided you're both ready, willing, and lubricated.

Exploring new locations on the body for titillation can also prove quite satisfying. Don't go directly for the genitals or breasts immediately.

Excite different sensations by teasing other erogenous zones with caresses or kisses. Here are some you'll want to explore:

The Arms and Hands

A kiss upon the back of the hand or a fingertip swirled around the palm and stroked along the wrist is nice. Four fingertips dragged slowly up the length of the underside of the entire arm is nicer still.

The Shoulders

Stroking and kneading them can help increase blood flow and decrease stress. Soft licks and kisses across them can increase arousal.

The Neck

The neck serves as the passageway from the head to the heart, and when properly stimulated can open up. It also provides a fine bridge between the mouth and breasts. Start with gentle strokes and licks along the muscles at the sides of the neck, adjusting your pressure depending on your lover's response. The back of the neck is also quite responsive to light touch.

The Earlobes

Packed with nerve endings, the earlobes rank as a sensual delicacy. Tickle them with your fingers or tongue, kiss or lick them. Try pressing around the rim of the ear.

The Forehead and Scalp

Caresses here bring you close to your partner's main sex organ, the brain. Stroking and kissing the forehead can ease a lover's stress, bringing about the kind of relaxation that creates openness to sexual activity. Short fingertip strokes across the scalp can also turn a "not-tonight-dear headache" into a request for more.

The Feet

Start by cleaning them in a warm tub, drying, then rubbing lotion or olive oil into each nook and cranny. Foot massage is an art unto itself, as a reflexologist will tell you. With practice, however, you can master enough simple techniques to satisfy your lover. Try long strokes on the instep for starters, and some thumb kneading on the front base of the arch. Gently twirl each toe between your thumb and forefinger, then move a finger into the particularly sensitive area in between each toe.

The Breasts

Suckling the nipple comes naturally to human beings. As such, nipples receive most (sometimes all) of the attention during sex play. Indeed, they are the most sensitive part of the breast, and seem to be directly connected to the genitals. But there's far more to the breasts in terms of sensual possibility. In fact, most women prefer having the rest of their breasts stroked and stimulated prior to nipple play. The undersides of the breasts are especially neglected and appreciative of attention. In fact, lavish attention on the entire breast besides the nipple area. Save that area for last.

From Location to Sensation

Now that you've found some new sweet spots on your lover's body to titillate, try these techniques: Drag your hair across your lover's skin. Long hair works best, but even a buzz cut provides wondrous new feelings. Your partner may even giggle because your hair is tickling him or her. Nothing's wrong with that. In fact, alternate your hair and fingertips for a tickle fest. Laughter is a marvelous aphrodisiac.

A soft paintbrush dragged across the body can make your lover feel like a work of art. Vary the length, pressure and location of your

Question: I've been married for ten years and my partner doesn't respond to my old seduction techniques. Do you have any ideas for new approaches?

There are as many ways to seduce as there are lovers. If your partner isn't responding, perhaps he or she needs something different now than before. Take the time to focus on your partner and consider what that might be. The best seduction strategies are specific to the intended. To get you thinking, here are some approaches that tend to be successful:

- Extend the invitation. An artful, thoughtful invitation to sex proves irresistible to many, especially romantic types.
- Pour on the charm. Charm makes people forget their

insecurities and feel desirable— as well as desire for the charmer.

- Feign Indifference. Strange as it seems, many of us become excited when our mate appears focused on something besides us. So pour your focus into something you enjoy. Or tease your lover, telling him or her, "Not now, but in a little while, perhaps."
- Take the side road. Some couples find a direct "let's fuck" sexy as hell. Others need more subtlety. If your partner is among them, consider artful ways to advance your cause without spelling it out in neon lights. Men, take her out to dinner and use the rose you brought her to stroke her thigh under the table. Tell her she looks almost as beautiful in that dress as she did last time you were in bed. Women, tell him how handsome he looks when he's relaxed and that you know just how to relax him.
- Sit down for a soulful chat. Have nothing more on your agenda than intimate talk and maybe a little cuddling. If you let go of expectations about how the evening will end, and share for the sake of just being together, passion may arise naturally.
- Do something special for your partner. Guiding your mate through a new experience he or she has wanted to try can lead to a powerful state of arousal.
- Pamper away. Doing kind things unto your lover's body will often get him or her to do the same unto you.
- Get away from it all. Experiencing something new that wakes up all the senses. So try planning an erotic getaway in a place sure to stir your partner's sense of fun and well being.

strokes for maximum titillation. Paint brushes—the kind you'll find in an art store—provide the most sensitive touch; you can perform an on-site test by brushing each small brush in the store across the back of your hand. Feather dusters are also great for sex play. Just make sure that the brushes and dusters are new, and reserved for this purpose only. Flavored, edible gels, lotions and honey dust can sweeten oral play. Spread them onto different parts of your bodies and lick each other clean. (Make sure to read the labels to insure that each substance is safe and won't irritate the delicate skin of the mouth or genitals.)

Temperature contrasts can lead to especially intense effects. Many lotions can be heated before application. Just be sure to apply with your hand to make sure they're not too hot, especially for sensitive genitals, which are more heat sensitive than your fingers. Also look for "warming oils" that heat up when you apply and blow on them. Alternately, try ice cubes—but only with your partner's approval.

If you'd like to see a visual presentation of the material in this chapter, refer to the following videos from the Sinclair Intimacy Institute Video Library: *Discovering Unforgettable Sex,* Volume 3: *The Art of Seduction,* and *Dr. Sandra Scantling's Ordinary Couples, Extraordinary Sex,* Volume 3: *Keeping Sex Extraordinary.*

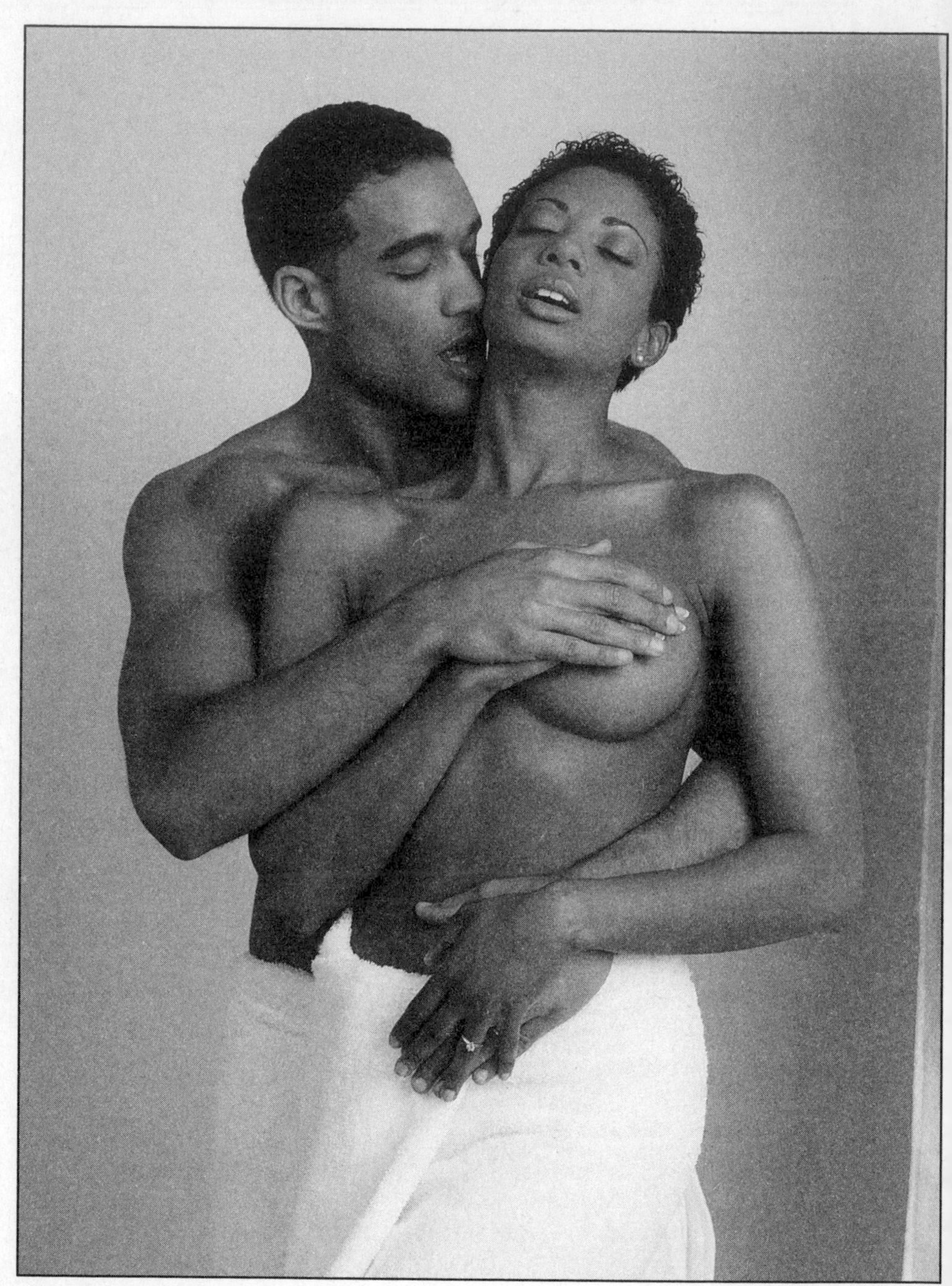

Secret #4

Lover, Know Yourself

> *The intimacy in sex is never only physical. In a sexual relationship, we may discover who we are in ways otherwise unavailable to us, and at the same time we allow our partner to see and know that individual. As we unveil our bodies, we also disclose our persons.*
>
> —Dr. Thomas Moore
> *Soul Mates*

Much of the initial education we receive about sexuality comes from peers (who may be seriously misinformed), parents who are embarrassed to discuss it (and may have some serious inhibitions themselves), overzealous (and sometimes hypocritical) men of the cloth, and/or erotic magazines like Playboy or Hustler. As a result, many of us remain underinformed, confused and even slightly ashamed of our sexual organs. Think back upon how you learned the names of each of your body parts. You probably learned an accurate name for each, except for your genitals. What message did that give you? That they're different? That they're dirty?

To make matters worse, we've been living with these distorted ideas about sexuality for so long, we no longer recognize that they are there. And that means that they can continue to interfere with our sexual self-image, as well as our sexual pleasure.

Fortunately, good, healthy sex with a loving partner can go a long way toward helping you accept, enjoy and celebrate your sexual self. Once you intimately explore your own body and discover its potential for pleasure, you may find yourself that what shamed you before is actually a wonderful, miraculous part of you.

The Female Genitalia: A Guided Tour for Women

Since a woman's sexual organs are primarily internal, it is possible to go through most of your life without ever really becoming acquainted with them. That would be a shame. As they say, knowledge is power. If you want to feel sexually self-confident, you need to make the acquaintance of your sexual self. That means setting aside time for yourself to explore what you've been given at birth and to find the kind of stimulation you find most pleasurable.

Before reading on, you might want to find a private place where you can undress and spread your legs open in front of a mirror. (A handheld mirror should work fine.) Don't be surprised at how your genitals look, if you've never seen them in a mirror before. As you read about each part, gently touch it and test out some of the stimulation techniques. This will help you become more comfortable with your sexual organs and more informed about the kind of stimulation that works for you.

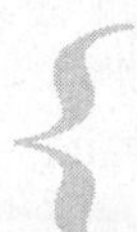

Tip: *Some women are embarrassed to look at or touch their genitals because they consider them "dirty." That's a myth. A clean vagina is thought to contain fewer germs than the average mouth.*

The Vaginal Area Pleasure Centers

The vulva, the term that refers to a woman's external genitals, includes the mons, labia, clitoris and the perineum. All of these areas are sensitive to pleasure. When you look at the vulva, the first thing you're likely to notice is the triangle of pubic hair sitting atop your genital region. Underneath rests a palm-sized pad known as the mons (or mons veneris after the Roman goddess of love). This soft, fleshy mound protects the pubic bone during the hard thrusting of intercourse. It contains many nerve endings. Some women enjoy touch or pressure here, especially before or during intercourse. Cup it in your palm and softly squeeze or vibrate your hand. That should feel pretty good.

Bring your vaginal lips between your thumb and forefinger and try massaging or lightly pulling them. Try moving your hand all around with the outer lips, as you clasp them gently between your thumb and forefinger. Then try using the thumbs on both hands. You may be surprised at how good this feels.

Next, part the labia majora. Trace a wetted finger around the lips, pausing to experience what that feels like. Go over the areas where touch feels best.

The clitoris, covered by the clitoral hood, sits at the crest of the labia minora where the two lips meet. Sex researchers know that the clitoris is vital to the female orgasm. It is incredibly sensitive to the touch. This remarkable little organ consists of a tiny rounded head (or glans) and lengthy shaft. Though the entire clitoral system is actually similar in size (and function) to the penis, most of it is hidden inside the body. Only the glans and a tiny fraction of the shaft are visible. And you may have to squint to see even that—the head of the average clitoris is no larger than a pearl, which makes its power all the more remarkable. Its only function is to provide sexual pleasure. (Unfortunately, parents rarely speak about the clitoris when they talk to their children about sex.)

When a woman becomes aroused, the glans and the shaft of the clitoris fill with blood and may swell (some even double in diameter). As erotic stimulation continues, the clitoris becomes extremely sensitive and the tissues of the clitoral hood swell to cover and protect it.

Due to the region's hypersensitivity, many women prefer indirect rather than direct clitoral stimulation. For these women, licking or stroking the labia minora near the clitoris can prove more pleasurable.

On the other hand, there are some women who love direct clitoral stimulation. Try gently—so gently, you barely feel as if you're touching it—by passing a fingertip over the clitoral hood, then parting the hood and stroking the clitoris. It may take a moment to find the exact spot, but don't worry—you will.

Although the word "vagina" is often mistakenly applied to the entire female genital region, the term actually applies specifically to the birth canal, the corridor in which a man inserts his penis for intercourse.

The vagina begins at the vaginal opening and continues inward for several inches, ending at the cervix or neck of the womb. Most of the nerve endings in the vagina occur over its first third, though some women also report pleasurable sensations from pressure deeper within.

A lesser-know pleasure spot is the perineum, the area of skin located between the anus and the vaginal opening. This little strip is rich in nerve endings. Stroking it can enhance sexual arousal. Just make sure to first apply a light, water-based lubricant so that you experience pleasure rather than friction on this delicate area.

Inside the vagina is the "G-spot," or Grafenberg-spot," an area that serves as a source of great pleasure for many women. The location of this coin-sized, raised area of sensitivity may vary, but it is typically about three inches into the vagina underneath the surface of the front wall. The "G-spot" is relatively hard for a woman to reach on her own but can be stimulated with the help of a sex toy or a partner's fingers. (See Chapter 6 for more information on the "G-spot.")

Male Genitalia: A Guided Tour for Men

The structure of the male genitalia is much more obvious. The penis basically consists of a head (also called the glans) and a shaft or body. On uncircumcised males, a fleshy hood called a foreskin covers the head. It can be easily rolled back to expose the glans.

The entire penis is sensitive to touch, particularly during sexual arousal when the organ fills with blood, swells and points upward. This is typically called "an erection." The head, however, houses a particularly high concentration of nerve endings, making it so sensitive that many men prefer no more than a light touch there. The shaft is another pleasure zone. A hand grasped around the shaft and stroked its entire length again and again, with pressure emphasized in different areas depending on preference, is the most common and effective form of manually stimulating the penis. Two other highly pleasurable spots include the coronal ridge—the rim that separates the head from the shaft—and the thin strip of skin on the underside of the head called the frenulum. Gentle, searching finger strokes should tell you exactly where these little treasures are hiding.

Tip: *Men, if you're wondering whether your equipment measures up, consider these facts:*

The average length of an erect penis is around five to six inches. Almost all of the vagina's nerve endings occur within an inch or two of the vaginal opening. If you do the math, you realize that even a penis well below average in length will be more than adequate to effectively stimulate a vagina. Sex therapists report that the vast majority of women who complain about their partner's penis size are those who consider their partner's penis too large for comfort.

An often-ignored area of sensitivity is the scrotum—the pouch of skin underneath the penis that encloses the testicles. Some men enjoy a soft, cupping massage of the scrotum. The testicles—small hard orbs about the size of grapes floating within the scrotum—are highly sensitive, and must be handled very gently.

Men also have a perineum. This sensitive strip of skin is located just below the base of the scrotum and runs to the top of the anus. Many men will find stroking the perineum with a lightly lubricated finger very pleasurable.

Why It's Essential to Discover and Assert Your Sexual Boundaries

Exploring your body will give you a good idea of what you like, how you like it—and what you definitely don't like. It's important for each of you to be honest with yourself first, and then with each other, about what you don't like—whether it's being approached for sex in a certain way, having your lover use a certain kind of touch, or engaging in a specific sexual act. If you find your lover's touch too rough, or not fast enough, say something. Honor yourself, and your preferences. Anything short of that is dishonest, and a barrier to true intimacy.

Realize, too, that it's your job to make your likes and dislikes clear. Don't expect your partner to understand intuitively. It's not fair to expect anyone to read your mind.

To communicate your needs without making your partner feel belittled, try positive statements, such as, "I love it when you touch me there," or "It feels so much better when you use less pressure on that area." Making pleasurable sounds or sighing "yes" when your lover gets it right can be very encouraging.

If your lover continues to miss the mark, show rather than tell. Trace your own fingers over your favorite places on your body using the techniques and pressures you find most stimulating. Leading by example is often the most powerful tutorial. Good communication is essential to good sex. Yet it doesn't always have to be verbal. If you feel shy about indicating your preferences, remember that most people find a partner who knows what he or she likes and can express this, quite sexy.

Releasing Unhealthy Sexual Inhibitions

Any sexual relationship may eventually bump into—and maybe even crash and burn against—the sexual inhibitions of one or both partners. The sexual attitudes of one's parents, pastor, or culture may be exerting a subtle—or not so subtle—influence that makes it difficult to freely express your sexuality with each other. If you have negative feelings about sex, or certain sexual acts, try to explore how or where they originated. What were your parents' attitudes toward sex? How do they color your sexual outlook today? Did a classmate publicly or even privately humiliate you over a sexual matter? Has anyone been inappropriately sexual with you? As a child? As a teenager? Did you feel rejected by people of the opposite sex when you entered the dating years? If you are religious, what is your perception of your church's teachings on sex?

You might want to do some writing on the subject so that you can see the content of your own mind. If you have negative feelings about sex, or consider it "unholy" or consider yourself unattractive or unworthy of pleasure, your attitudes will create a barrier to real intimacy, and ultimately, your own satisfaction. They will also prevent your partner from experiencing fulfillment in physical love. That's why it's worth exploring this sometimes painful area and finding your way to come out on the other side of it. Here are possible ways you might want to approach this. Choose the one that's right for you:

- Enlist your partner in the cause. Inhibitions limit intimacy and create mistrust between lovers. Reverse the downward slide by discussing the inhibition with your partner and asking for his or her help in defining and overcoming it. Apologize for past problems caused by the inhibition and assert your determination to conquer it. Ask for advice, help and counsel.

- During intimacy, focus on your sensations, not your thoughts. If you find yourself having negative thoughts about your body, or the sexual act itself, observe them but let them pass. Make a promise to yourself that you will make time later to work through those thoughts.

- Say "no" when you want to, without feeling ashamed. Having sex because you would feel guilty not to can be as emotionally damaging as letting guilt prevent you from having sex. Respect yourself and your body.

- Apply humor. Diffuse the negative emotions that build up around inhibitions by enjoying a good laugh about yourself. Instead of gnashing your teeth and emotionally beating yourself up, think of how ridiculous it is to let bad ideas stand between you and your fulfillment. Laughter puts inhibitions in their proper perspective.

• Make your partner feel better. Praising and delighting in your partner can help your mate feel better about his or her body, help you feel better about your body and help both of you feel better about sex. It also sets you up for a nice payback.

• Bathe before sex, if you are afraid your genitals won't smell good to your partner. If that thought tends to make you tense during oral sex, ask your partner how you smell. If you've bathed just before sex, it shouldn't be a problem. Your lover may love your scent. Your fear may have no basis in fact.

Conquering an inhibition can take a little doing. Understand that you may struggle and slip back occasionally, but that it will get easier as old patterns are broken and new satisfactions are discovered. But, it's a worthwhile journey. Freeing yourself from any sexual inhibitions will not only boost your confidence, and make you even sexier to your partner, but it may also free up energy for other areas of your life. No doubt your partner will appreciate the new, more sexually confident you.

DEMYTHOLOGIZING MASTURBATION

Despite some nasty myths about masturbation, the truth is that self-stimulation offers an excellent, risk-free way to become more comfortable with your sexuality, as well as more knowledgeable about your sexual needs. Bringing yourself to orgasm is a great stress-reliever, too. A recent national study indicates that 95 percent of men and 89 percent of women masturbate. Individuals who have a regular sexual partner report higher rates of masturbation. That's probably because they tend to focus more on sexual activity, since they are already enjoying it in their relationship.

To enjoy this activity, choose a place and hour of day when you won't be interrupted. If you live with others, you may want to run the tub and lock the bathroom door. If the idea of pleasuring yourself makes you uncomfortable, take some deep breaths. Relax as much as you can. Concentrate on all the wonderful sensations flowing through your body. In this state, you should find the experience pleasant and informative.

Feeling Good About Your Body

Individuals who consider themselves unattractive in any way, or otherwise deficient (perhaps considering their breasts or penis "too small," or their belly and backside too large), may feel so self-conscious about being naked in front of their partner that it takes away from their ability to give themselves freely in sex.

The truth is you don't have to be a supermodel or Hollywood hunk to be a great lover, or remain attractive to your partner. The most important thing is to learn to feel good about yourself. The way you feel about yourself will radiate out to others. People will treat you accordingly. There have always been women—and men—who aren't great "lookers," but they're still magnetic to the opposite sex. These are people who are very comfortable with their sexuality, and themselves; they take good care of their bodies, and they know how to dress themselves to make the most of their strong points. Their appeal has nothing to do with what Nature gave them, but with what they have made of themselves.

Artificial Lubrication Can Make a Big Difference

Most women's vaginas naturally lubricate when they become aroused. But the amount of lubrication they generate varies widely—depending on the woman, the situation, the stage of her menstrual cycle and/or her age. Using a water-based lubricant can help make manual stimulation and intercourse more comfortable and arousing. There are many different kinds on the market. Here's what to consider when choosing a lubricant:

- Water-based vs. Oil-based. Oil-based lubricants can cling to the walls of the vagina for days, which could lead to yeast and bacterial problems. Oil-based lubricants can also degrade latex so avoid using them with latex products such as condoms or latex toys. Another problem: they often leave stains on clothes and sheets. This is why most experts recommend water-based lubricants, even though they dry out more quickly.

- Thin vs. Thick. Consistency is largely a matter of personal preference. Thinner lubes tend to be good for clitoral stimulation, thin or medium ones work nicely for vaginal play, and thicker products may prove useful for anal exploration.

- Silicone. These lubricants are designed to stay slippery in

If you want to follow their lead, begin by accepting yourself exactly as you are. Even if there are things about you you'd like to change, extend to yourself the same unconditional regard you'd want from the people who love you most. If you find this difficult, find a good therapist

water, making them useful in a hot tub or shower. They're long lasting and won't dry up like water-based lubricants, but you'll need to use soap to wash them off.

- Flavored vs. Taste/Odor Free. Most couples stick to neutral lubes. Flavored lubricants provide a fun change of pace for couples who want to add a little sweetness to their oral play. However, both partners should make sure they're not allergic to any of the taste-enhancing ingredients.
- Variety Packs. Many companies sell sample-sized collections of all their lubricant products. These samplers provide couples with an economical way to test out a number of different lubes.

Women, be careful with lubricants that contain glycerin and the spermicide nonoxynol-9, both of which can irritate the vagina. Glycerin, a form of sugar, is a very common ingredient in sweet-tasting lubricants and may cause problems for women prone to yeast infections. The spermicide Nonoxynol-9 was once widely recommended by health experts because it was falsely believed to kill HIV in laboratory tests. Unfortunately, this detergent-like compound has turned out to be less reliable in the bedroom. Besides providing a false sense of security, nonoxynol-9 can cause irritation and microtears in the mucous membranes of the vagina and anus—actually making some people more vulnerable to HIV and other sexually transmitted diseases.

who can model unconditional self-regard for you. Learning to love yourself as you are is a priceless gift. That's not to say that you should give up efforts at constructive change. It's just that it's easier to make those changes when you like yourself, than when you reject some part of yourself.

Learning to Orgasm: Guidance for Women

There is a lot of misinformation in circulation about the female orgasm. Scenes in movies show women climaxing almost instantly, as if all that were necessary was a swell of romantic music on the soundtrack. Photos in many print ads imply that just a whiff of the right cologne will send a woman to the brink. This sort of nonsense leaves many real women and their partners feeling inadequate.

The truth is, most female orgasms require time, technique and effort. And all that can fall short, too. Even some of the most orgasmic women are unable to climax every time. And some have trouble doing it at all. According to a study in the Journal of the American Medical Association, between 22 and 28 percent of women reported that they are unable to reach orgasm during sex.

The good news is that almost every woman can achieve sexual climax. It's not that complicated. It just takes time and practice. If you're having trouble achieving orgasm, try this step-by-step program, designed by Joseph LoPiccolo, Ph.D., and Julia R. Heiman, Ph.D., authors of *Becoming Orgasmic: A Sexual and Personal Growth Program for Women.* Take your time, staying as long as it takes on one step before moving on to the next. And don't get discouraged. It takes practice and perseverance to learn anything new. The effort may be great. But your reward for learning to orgasm will be a lot more pleasurable than any diploma. You may also benefit from watching the Sinclair Video Library video *Becoming Orgasmic*, which shows a couple learning these techniques for achieving female climax for the first time.

Here is a summary of the steps in the LoPiccolo and Heiman book:

• Review the sections on female anatomy and releasing inhibitions earlier in this chapter. Oftentimes, an inability to achieve orgasm stems from feelings of guilt, anxiety or a simple lack of know-how.

• Stop setting orgasm as your goal. Give yourself a period of time—say four to six weeks—just to enjoy yourself without worrying about a goal.

• Learn to treat yourself like a queen. Take a long bubble bath.

• Dress up in something that makes you feel sexy and powerful. Dim the lights. Put on some music. Stand in front of a full-length mirror and congratulate yourself on everything regal and fabulous about you. Explore your beauty and the pleasure of your own touch.

• Get acquainted with your genitals. Use a hand-mirror and the anatomy notes in the beginning of this chapter as your guide. Remember that the clitoris is one key to orgasm, but there are other areas that will help push you closer. Experiment with different strokes, rhythms, and intensities. Make circles with your fingers. Notice what feels good.

• Connect your mind and your groin. Orgasms require cooperation between the brain and genitals. Get them on the same page through relaxation and meditation. Start with deep breathing, feeling the breath move throughout your body. Feel it flow from your head to your groin. Once your mind is clear, guide it into creating sexy thoughts or images. Many women enjoy and require fantasies or erotic material in order to stimulate themselves, so feel free to entertain any thoughts you want. (See Chapter 9 for more on fantasies.) Touch your genitals and your nipples and other erogenous zones while you fantasize. Don't try to orgasm, just enjoy yourself.

• Role-play orgasm. When you're comfortable touching yourself, and you're becoming aroused, fake an orgasm. Imagine what an orgasm might look, sound and feel like and then practice one. Yell, pant, moan, twitch, curl your toes. Be really loud and dramatic about it. This might feel silly, but for many women pretending to have an orgasm can help break down subconscious barriers and open the door to a real orgasm.

• Orgasm triggers are little tricks women can use as they approach climax to push themselves over the edge. Some women hold their breath and tense up. Some curl their toes. Some arch their backs. Some conjure up a particularly erotic image. Notice what's happening in your body as you touch yourself. And try out these triggers and see what they do for you.

• Learn to read the signs. Some women describe the feeling of orgasm as a wave of intense pleasure. Some describe a "fluttery feeling" that happens as the muscles around the vagina and uterus undergo a series of contractions. Every woman feels an orgasm differently and orgasms often vary in intensity from one time to the next. Your first orgasm may be so subtle that you may not even be sure that it actually happened. Keep exploring. If you feel relaxed and happy after stimulation, you're onto something.

• If after several weeks of manual stimulation, you don't feel like you're making progress (or if you've had orgasms and are ready for some new sensations), then try a vibrator. Many preorgasmic women find the intense, regular rhythms of a vibrator can stimulate them to their first orgasm. (See Chapter 7 for more details about what to use and where to buy).

• Don't push, just let it happen. Achieving orgasm is not so much a logical, straight-line process as the setting up of an environment in which one can occur. Think of it more as a thunderstorm waiting to happen. Set yourself up in the right time, place and conditions, and the clouds will eventually break and make you deliriously soaked.

Safe Sex for Committed Partners

Few lovers love condoms, but they do have their advantages. They are considered an effective form of birth control, they offer some protection against sexually transmitted disease, and can also be used to sheath sex toys such as vibrators and dildos, to keep them at their hygienic best.

Choosing the kind that's right for you, however, isn't always easy. How do you know which material is better, whether to get the lubricated kind or the nonlubricated kind, the plain or the "pleasure-ribbed?"

Here is some information that can help.

- Go for latex unless you and your partner have latex allergies. (Allergies can develop in people who are frequently exposed to latex, and may cause rashes, nausea and even dangerous respiratory problems.) Polyurethane condoms are the condom of choice for the latex-sensitive. They're thinner than latex , and safe to use with oil-based lubricants, but they break more easily. Lambskin provides a more natural feel, but they are unreliable as barriers against viruses such as HIV.

- Do not store condoms in wallets, glove compartments, refrigerators or anywhere else where they might be exposed to temperature extremes or moisture. Bright light can also lead to degradation. Keep an eye on the expiration date printed on the packaging, and err on the side of caution, especially if the wrapper looks or feels worn. Condoms that are stored properly are good for about three to five years.

- If you choose lubricated condoms, beware of those coated with the spermicide nonoxynol-9. While this may provide some extra protection against unwanted pregnancy, nonoxynol-9 can be very irritating for sensitive individuals. Condoms with water-based lubricants or silicone lubricants are a better bet.
- Experiment with size. Some men prefer the snugger fit of smaller sizes, while others will enjoy the extra room afforded by large varieties. Also experiment with shape. Your options include condoms that advertise themselves as straight, flared, indented or designed with extra room for the head of the penis. Reservoir-tip condoms designed to hold sperm after ejaculation are becoming increasingly common.
- Condom breakage is often the result of air trapped inside the condom. To reduce air bubbles, pinch the end of the condom with one hand as you roll it on with the other and carefully drain out any air bubbles that you find along the way.

If you want to experiment with ribbed or colored condoms, look for those made by an established manufacturer rather than an upstart. You want to buy from a company that has satisfied customers for years, instead of one that hasn't yet proven itself.

Sharing Your New Skill

Once you've learned how to climax by yourself and you've spent enough time enjoying the experience for yourself, you may want to share this treasure with your partner. For some, the transition will be easy. But many women may not orgasm right away with their partners, and some never do. To help ease into it, concentrate on increasing feelings of sensuality, pleasure and intimacy.

Take at least a few weeks to build trust and technique. You may see results faster if you concentrate on the techniques below and forego intercourse during this time.

- Reacquaint yourselves with whole-body sensation by giving each other non-sexual massages. Taking turns giving and receiving. Offer each other feedback after each session. Begin your next sessions with touches and strokes that are informed by what you're learning.

- Once you're getting aware of your sensation preferences, you may want to try masturbating in front of each other. There's no need to worry if you can't bring yourself to orgasm. This is a big step and many partners are a little nervous at first. After couples get used to the idea, however, it can be a huge turn-on.

- When you're both comfortable with individual masturbation and ready to progress further, teach your partner to help you masturbate. Use your hand to guide him to your pleasure spots. Tell him how and where you like to be touched. Don't attempt to orgasm this time, just let yourself feel his touch while you communicate your preferences. Neither partner should feel any pressure to perform—just relax, communicate and explore.

• Keep practicing your mutual pleasure sessions, and when you've been able to achieve orgasm with his help, engage in intercourse with the aid of manual stimulation. Stimulate your clitoris while his penis is inside you. Some positions are better than others for this, so keep experimenting around until you find one that works. (See Chapter 5 for ideas.)

• Keep stimulating yourself and concentrating on your own pleasure. Be present with yourself and aware of the sensations in your body. Notice how little moves or variations in posture can enhance pleasure.

• Try alternate activities. Orgasms happen in all sorts of ways, and no one way is better than another. Have your partner perform oral sex on you. (See Chapter 10.) Have your partner manually stimulate you while you play with your breasts. Manually stimulate yourself while your partner pleasures the rest of your body. Use a sex toy to stimulate yourself during intercourse.

• Keep your eyes off the prize. Instead of focusing on orgasm, immerse yourself in all the wonderful sensations you're experiencing. Try different combinations of genital and body stimulation with increasing pleasure as your goal. Feel the joy and sensations running throughout your body, and before you know it, an orgasm may just drop into your lap.

MUTUAL MASTURBATION EXERCISE

A game of "Show, Tell and Touch" is an excellent way for lovers to set boundaries, demonstrate preferences, overcome inhibitions, and make a quantum leap in satisfaction.

To start, both of you need to strip naked and find a comfortable place—such as a bed or bathtub—where you can observe one another. Take turns talking about your bodies—your erogenous zones, what you like, where you like it, the order of stimulation you prefer. Also, discuss your discomforts. Point out your boundaries—areas you don't like being touched and actions that turn you off. Go over your entire body. Let your partner touch you, following your lead.

Resist the urge to segue into full-fledged sex. This exercise is meant to help you get comfortable with one another, and make later sexual encounters more pleasurable. If you skimp here because you're so turned on you want to consummate your love, the next lovemaking session may not be any better.

Play this game several times—at different times—to make sure that you and your partner have time to absorb all the information.

Question: I know I should wear a condom, but stopping to put it on really ruins the mood just as things are heating up. What should my partner and I do?

Couples often dread putting on condoms because a man can lose his erection in the process. To help a man keep his erection, his partner can lick, stroke and caress him as he applies the condom. Or she can put it on herself, slowly rolling it over his penis as she stares expectantly into his eyes. Once the condom is secure, she can continue to pleasure him manually (especially if it's a lubricated condom) or orally if it's not. Try making little circles around the head of the penis.

Men: Overcoming Common Sexual Challenges

Premature or rapid ejaculation can be a major source of embarrassment and stress for both men and their partners. A lack or ejaculatory control (commonly referred to as "climaxing too quickly") is a common problem among men of all ages and socioeconomic groups, but it tends to be most prevalent among young men.

It doesn't need to be an ongoing problem, however. There are steps you can take to improve ejaculatory control. The process involves training yourself to recognize the sensations that lead up to that point of "ejaculatory inevitability," then using specific techniques to delay the orgasm.

Many men try to control premature ejaculation by distracting themselves from the sensation. They try to think about a sport they love, a situation at work, unpleasant co-workers—anything besides sex. This technique may work for some. But therapists have found that the best way to delay ejaculation is not through distraction, but by being super-focused on the moment. If you are present enough to the sensations, and learn to recognize those that accompany impending orgasm, you can suspend or lighten the stimulation until the urge has subsided.

The concept of focusing on the sensations leading to orgasm, rather than attempting to distract yourself, comes from the work of Dr. J. Semens in the 1950s. His work has since been modified by sex therapists, including the sex therapy pioneers William H. Masters, M.D., and Virginia E. Johnson.

Some therapists suspect that the way men learn to masturbate during adolescence (bringing on orgasm rapidly so they don't get caught) contributes to the problem. Fortunately, masturbation also offers a great way to retrain yourself. Masturbate to the point just before ejaculatory inevitability, stop your strokes until the urge passes, then restart. Repeat this process several times. Delay your orgasms longer and longer until you're confident of your ejaculatory control.

While most men can improve their ejaculatory control through practicing these simple techniques, not all men can. If those techniques don't work for you, ask your family doctor for a referral to a urologist, or contact the American Association of Sex Educators, Counselors and Therapists. (The web address is www.aasect.org)

IMPOTENCE: ADVICE FOR MEN

Temporary bouts of erectile dysfunction will affect just about every man at some time in his life. So don't be alarmed if you fail to achieve an erection once or twice. Try getting more exercise, making sure you get a full night's sleep and eliminating fatty, cholesterol-building foods from your diet. Try to reduce the stress in your life. If you still find that you frequently have difficulty getting or sustaining an erection, do the manly thing and get help. See a urologist. The symptoms may signal a more serious health problem.

You may have a physical condition that's contributing to the problem, or such an overload of stress that your body has little energy for anything but essential functions. There are many physical, environmental, and psychological factors that can contribute to erectile dysfunction, including pollutants, clogged arteries, job stress, many prescription medications, smoking, heavy drinking, or unresolved feelings toward your partner. Whatever the cause, a urologist who specializes in treating male sexual dysfunction can help you sort it out. Your doctor may also refer you to a therapist who specializes in treating sexual health. Don't cheat yourself out of a good sex life by covering up the problem, out of shame. Erection problems are very common. Fortunately, erectile dysfunction is curable in the vast majority of men.

Tip: *Many prescription medications can cause erection problems. These include certain: high blood pressure medicines, ulcer medications, low blood sugar medications, and some antidepressants. Certain popular antidepressant or anti-anxiety medications such as Prozac and Zoloft have been found to lessen sexual feeling and inhibit orgasm in both men and women. Talk to your doctor about the possibility of switching to a medication that doesn't have sexual side effects. Whenever you receive a new prescription, ask about all of the potential side effects, including those that can affect your sexual health.*

If you'd like to see a visual presentation of the material in this chapter, refer to the following videos from the Sinclair Intimacy Institute Video Library: The Better Sex Video Series, Volumes 1 and 2: *Sexual Positions for Lovers*, and *Unlocking the Secrets of the G-spot.*

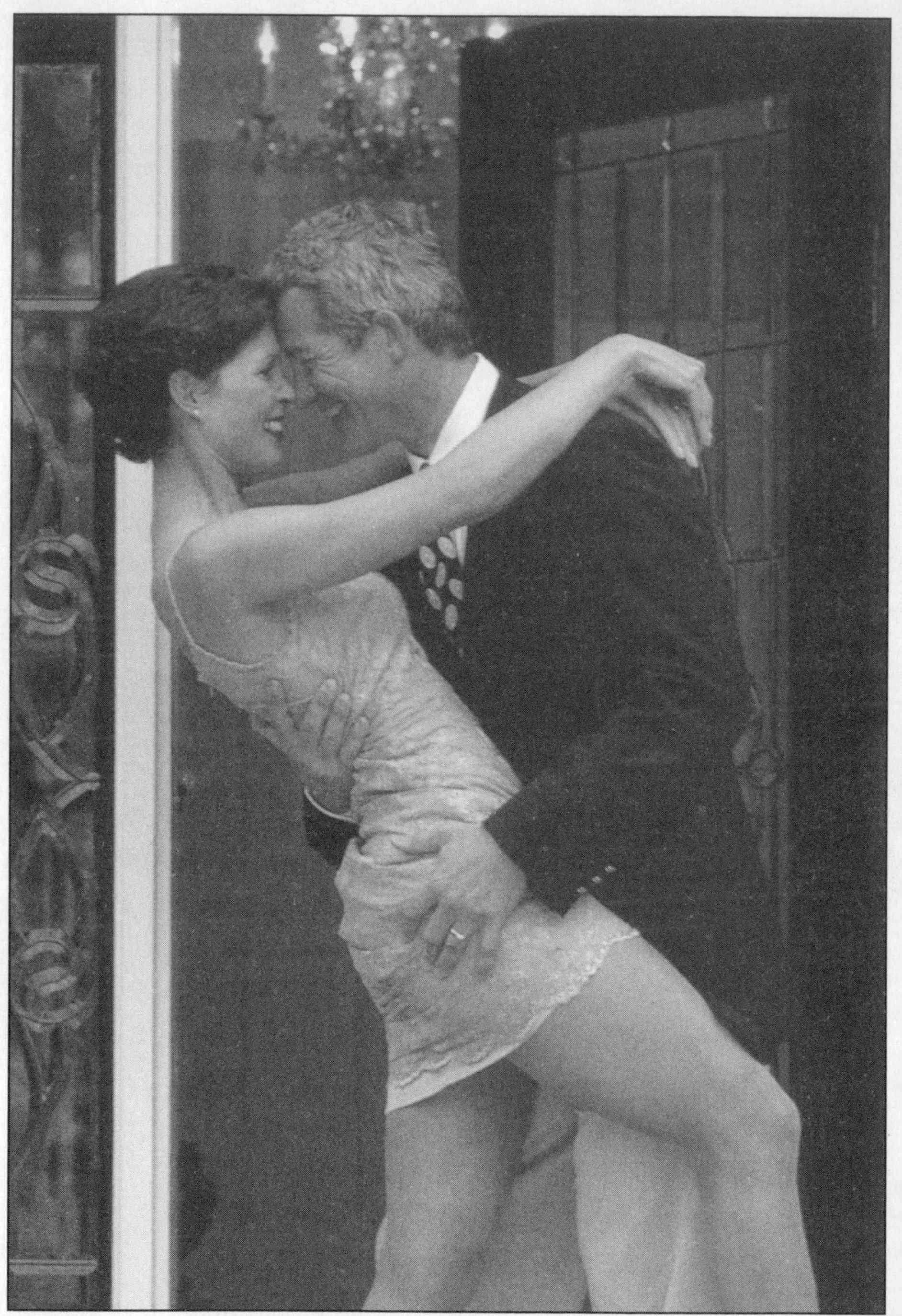

Secret #5

Position Yourself for Ultimate Pleasure

Sex is emotion in motion
—Mae West

Great sex partners develop like great dance duos. They start by mastering the basic moves. Then they work into advanced steps. From there, they improvise and experiment, developing their own moves and styles.

Couples who aren't enjoying great sex often lapse into stale routines. Early in their relationships, they fall into a rut that limits them to a basic position or two. After a while, instead of being spontaneous with each other, they just go through the motions.

By exploring new positions for intercourse and/or other erotic acts, you can keep sex fresh and interesting. Why not experiment with new ways to bring pleasure, taking advantage of the strengths of certain positions to bring you to the heights?

Positioning For Pleasure

Look at the Kama Sutra or another ancient erotic text, and you're struck by the variety of positions couples use. Most are variations of five basic positions familiar to almost everyone: the missionary, woman-on-top, rear entry, side-by-side and standing. By reviewing the basics and learning some of the variations, you can bring new excitement to your lovemaking.

The Missionary

This is sometimes known as "the matrimonial," and features the man on top. It was dubbed "the missionary position" in honor of Christian missionaries who tried to convince native cultures that it was the only moral position for intercourse. Where they got that idea, God only knows.

Whatever you call it, the position remains popular. The missionary is often the position that people use when they first experience intercourse. Many couples adopt it as their staple throughout their sex lives, and for good reason: it brings partners face to face, can effectively stimulate both, and is a good position from which to segue into other positions.

Still, many people think of man-on-top as old-fashioned, or as the "vanilla" of sexual postures—nice, but not terribly exciting. What they may not realize is that with a few subtle enhancements, the missionary position can offer some awesome new sensations.

The Clitoral Mission

Because the man seems to control much of the action, the missionary position is often associated with male pleasure. But with a few adjustments, this position can actually provide intense stimulation for the clitoris and "G-spot." Try these:

- **Riding High**. By propping himself on his arms and moving his groin up a few inches, the man can provide increased stimulation through contact between his pubic bone and the woman's vulva, especially the mons veneris.

- **Inside-Out.** This reversal of traditional leg arrangements finds the woman holding her legs together, while the man positions his legs on either side of hers. This adjustment moves the penis back and forth over the clitoris during penetration, increasing pleasure for both partners.

- **The Scissors.** The man kneels with one knee between the woman's thighs and his other leg stretched out to the side. The woman holds one of her legs down beneath his outstretched leg and curls the other around the hip of his inside leg. This creates full contact between the genitals, allowing for deep penetration and extra clitoral friction.

- **Using the Butt for Leverage.** By placing her hands on his buttocks and pulling herself up to meet her partner's strokes, the woman can increase the intensity of the position and guide the rhythm and angle of pressure so that it affords her maximum clitoral stimulation.

• **The Deep End.** By bending her legs, the woman opens herself and allows for deeper penetration. She can place her feet under her hips and rise up with her pelvis to gain greater leverage and control.

• **Arm Support.** By bending and bracing one leg, then angling his position so that he is supported by one arm, the man can thrust more powerfully and can use his free hand to stimulate his partner's erogenous zones.

• **Kneeling at the Altar.** By moving onto both knees, and placing himself between his partner's legs, the man can angle himself for deeper thrusting and "G-spot" stimulation. This can free up both hands for playing with the breast or providing other forms of stimulation. (The woman may want to use a pillow under her pelvis to enhance the angle.)

• **Stand and Deliver.** The man stands at the edge of the bed. The woman lies on the bed, positioning herself so he can thrust from a standing position. You may want to put pillows beneath her buttocks or something sturdy beneath his feet so that you join at the right height and the right angle for penetration.

• **Foot Rest**. With the man kneeling or standing, the woman bends her knees and places her feet flat against his chest. This can help her control depth and rhythm, and allow her to move her pelvis in an up-and-down rolling motion to rhythmically stimulate her "G-spot."

- **For the Flexible.** Women who enjoy good range of motion can bend their legs to the sides, or wrap them both around his waist, or extend them toward the ceiling, then drape them over his shoulders. These variations can offer excellent clitoral and "G-spot" stimulation. Women who have lower back problems should exercise caution. Go slowly at first, so you don't cramp up.

Woman-on-Top

Many women relish the woman-on-top or female superior position. Until recently, most women were taught to take a passive role during sex. The female superior position offers a chance to break out of that old, limiting stereotype. Because the woman controls the pace and angles, this position gives her a chance to establish what feels best to her. It also frees up a woman's hands to stimulate her clitoris, her breasts or her partner. And it's an excellent position for stimulating the "G-spot." Men usually enjoy this position every bit as much as women do. With her on top, the man can savor a great view of his loved one in enjoying her sexuality, even as he adds to her pleasure by stimulating her lips, neck, breasts and other erogenous zones. This position also gives a man a chance to catch his breath after the rigors of the missionary position. And because the stimulation of the woman-on-top position is usually less intense for the man, it can be a good way to control ejaculation and extend intercourse.

VARIETY-ON-TOP

Couples can vary the woman-on-top position depending on their preferences and flexibility. For instance:

• **Play All the Angles.** The woman can alter the stimulation through different postures—sitting straight up, leaning forward, or leaning backward. The man can also adjust his, sitting up, leaning back against a pillow, or lying down. He can also tilt his pelvis to vary stimulation. Go slowly as you adjust angles to avoid injury.

• **Back and Forth**. By placing his hands on her buttocks, the man can help work a back-and-forth motion into the usual up-and-down movement of this position, increasing clitoral and "G-spot" stimulation.

• **Holding Hands.** This move can aid balance and leverage, while also increasing intimacy.

• **Doing Squats.** By positioning herself in a squat position over her lover's penis, the woman can use the power of her legs to raise and lower herself, while giving the man room to meet her with his own thrusting motion.

• **On the Up and Up.** Men, don't just lie there and grin the whole time. To really drive your woman wild, try performing a series of short upward thrusts into her vagina. Some women report that this extra stimulation sends them over the edge into orgasm.

• **The Reverse-on-Top.** In this version, the man sits upright with his legs stretched in front of him. The woman turns her back to him, then kneels onto his penis. He circles her waist with his arms and thrusts from behind. In this position, she can raise and lower in response to his thrusts, and find the rhythm and angle that best stimulates her "G-spot."

Tip: *Sometimes, even a tiny change— like bending the legs, adjusting the angle of the pelvis, or changing the thrusting pattern from short, sharp strokes to long sensuous ones—can make a big difference. Making small adjustments to your favorite positions can be a good starting point for experimentation, especially if one of you is more comfortable sticking to the "tried and true."*

Rear Entry

Because most mammals engage exclusively in rear-entry (or doggie-style) intercourse, many men and women find that they can tap into their natural animal lust in this exciting pose. There are other benefits as well. For men, there's the great rear view. (Those who have a thing about a woman's behind love this.) The position is good for women, too, since it causes the man's penis to thrust against the front wall of the vagina where the "G-spot" is located.

Although rear-entry positions excel in deep vaginal and "G-spot" stimulation, they don't offer much in the way of clitoral excitement. What they do provide, though, is easy manual access to the clitoris. Couples can use their fingers or a vibrating toy on the clitoris and mons to increase sensation.

VARIATIONS ON REAR ENTRY

Prehistoric humans may have just stuck to the basics. But over time, people have developed a number of interesting variations on the primary rear-entry or "doggie-style" pose:

• **Standing Tall.** The woman kneels on the edge of the bed and the man enters her from behind while standing. This can lead to deeper, and more forceful, penetration.

• **The Reach Around.** The man can also enhance the pleasure of this position by reaching around his partner and placing a hand on her pelvis just above the pubic triangle, then pressing firmly but gently during thrusting to stimulate her "G-spot."

• **Rising to Meet Him.** The woman can deepen the stimulation by putting her head down and raising her buttocks. And for even deeper stimulation, she can arch her buttocks up into her partner's thrusts. Or she can reach back and hold hands with her partner to synchronize their movements and deepen the sense of intimacy.

• **Taking Control.** The woman can take control by moving her buttocks back and forth while the man remains still. This can help the woman customize the motion to her needs, while providing lots of pleasure to her man.

• **Full-Body Contact.** For a greater sense of intimacy, the woman can lie on her stomach while the man lies on top of her. This more nurturing variation allows for full-body contact and loving whispers.

Standing Postures

Because it can be pulled off almost anywhere, standing intercourse is often associated with quickies or illicit sexual encounters. Still, many couples find the position's physical intensity and emotional variety exciting even in their own bedrooms.

In the basic standing position, the woman leans back against a wall, with the man standing in front of her. The man cups his hands around her buttocks, positioning her pelvis as he enters. To aid in entry and in creating a favorable angle, the woman often wraps one leg around the man's hip or leg.

People with back problems or couples with big height differences may find the standing position difficult, or even painful. Everyone should go slowly at first, and make sure that both partners remain stable to avoid sudden shifts in weight that could lead to injury.

STANDING VARIATIONS

- **Lean On It.** To aid stability and ease the strain of the position, the woman can lean back against a wall, table or counter top for support. Just make sure the surface is comfortable and can accommodate the weight.

- **Trading Places.** Partners can switch places, with the man leaning back against the wall or table. The woman leans into him.

• **The Prop.** The woman props one foot up against a chair or other object to the side, allowing for easier entry and less strain.

• **Height adjustments.** Boots, high heels or bare feet can help even out height differences. One partner can also stand on something stable.

• **The Pick Up.** A man with good upper body strength, a sound lower back and cardiovascular endurance can hoist up his partner by locking his hands behind her buttocks and having her wrap her legs around him. For extra support, he can lean back against a wall. She can lock her hands behind his neck.

Side-by-Side

Side-by-side intercourse doesn't get as much attention as some of the more dramatic positions. But it remains a sweet, tender position that's very sensual. It can be especially useful for prolonged intercourse. It's also a nice choice for tired couples, as well as those who have back problems, arthritis or other physical challenges.

In the basic side-by-side position, partners lie on their sides facing each other, their legs gently intertwined. You may have to experiment a little with different angles and weight distributions. But intimacy is at a premium in this position, and both partners' hands are freed up for extra touching.

Tip: *Many couples are in the habit of letting one partner take the lead, with the other in a more passive role, during intercourse. If you find yourself in this mode, try switching roles. Changing roles allows both partners to explore a different side of their sexual selves. It can also lead to exciting new modes of stimulation—both physical and emotional. If one partner feels skeptical or nervous about the switch, discuss the idea. Use your imagination to make it fun and exciting for both of you.*

VARIATIONS ON THE SIDE

• **Left, Right, Left.** Instead of having the woman wrap both of her legs around the man, couples can "scissor" their legs with the man putting one of his legs on the outside, while the woman moves one of her legs inside. This can help redistribute weight and create new angles for clitoral stimulation.

• **The V.** By leaning away from each other (forming a "V" with their torsos) couples can tailor this pose for different angles of genital contact. The V can also help accommodate pregnant women, or partners carrying extra weight.

• **Spoons.** Basic side-by-side in reverse, with both partners facing the same direction. It's a gentle rear-entry position similar to the snuggling pose many couples use when they sleep. Women can enhance this posture by arching their lower backs and thrusting backwards into the man.

Gentle Positions for Special Needs

Couples with physical limitations such as back problems, arthritis, pregnancy, or chronic illness need to use extra care during intercourse. The side-by-side position offers a nice place to start. Changing positions several times during a single lovemaking session can also ease strain on specific body parts and muscles, while adding a variety of stimulation. Here are two other gentle postures for people with special needs. These can also be suitable for prolonged intercourse:

- **The X position.** This gentle variation of the female superior position can accommodate pregnant women or partners carrying extra weight. The posture sounds difficult, but in practice it's actually quite simple. The woman sits on the man and secures his penis inside of her. The couple then stretch out their legs and lean back on their arms, forming an X-shape. From there, they gently bump and grind.

- **Supporters.** An armless, padded chair can provide support for the back during sitting positions. The bottom partner can also slip a pillow behind the lower back for extra comfort. And a folded blanket can be used under the knees during reclining positions for lower-back support.

Simple Props for Enhancing Positions

Many objects around your house can turn a so-so position into a spectacular one. Just about anything can be adapted to sex play once you get your imagination rolling. Here are some ideas for starters:

• Pillows come in handy for angling the woman's pelvis for greater pleasure and for adjusting her height during various kneeling positions.

• Armless, padded chairs offer women great ease and rocking leverage for the female-superior position.

• A low-slung couch can allow both partners to use their feet for extra leverage and control.

• Carpeted stairs can provide an opportunity for a change of angle, height and pace. Be sure you have something to hang on to so you don't go tumbling down the stairs in the midst of ecstasy.

• The washing machine, the dining room table, the kitchen counter and other sturdy household surfaces can provide a support for height and weight redistribution during standing positions. Test them out first to make sure they're up to the task.

Pleasure Reading to Increase Your Repertoire

If you want to explore more positions, turn to some ancient Eastern texts on lovemaking that give examples (along with lyrical names) of different sexual positions. These texts also afford a philosophical glimpse into the history of sex and culture.

Books like the *Kama Sutra, The Ananga Ranga, The Perfumed Garden* and *The Teachings of the Tao* contain many simple positions, as well as some more complex or acrobatic poses for the adventurous.

Since the classic *Kama Sutra* was written for a male audience over 1500 years ago, some couples may prefer the more balanced and modern viewpoint of Anne Hooper's Kama Sutra, which was published in 1996.

As you're reading about new positions and gathering new material, remember that difficult poses aren't necessarily better. And just because a book recommends a pose doesn't mean that it will work for you, or that you can't adjust it to meet your needs. Couples should experiment and refine positions to accommodate their bodies and unique requirements. Ultimately, you will become your own teachers.

If you'd like to see a visual presentation of the material in this chapter, refer to the following videos from the Sinclair Intimacy Institute Video Library: The Better Sex Advanced Techniques, Volume 1: *Sexual Positions for Lovers: Beyond the Missionary, The Guide to Advanced Sexual Positions, Creative Positions for Lovers: Beyond the Bedroom.*

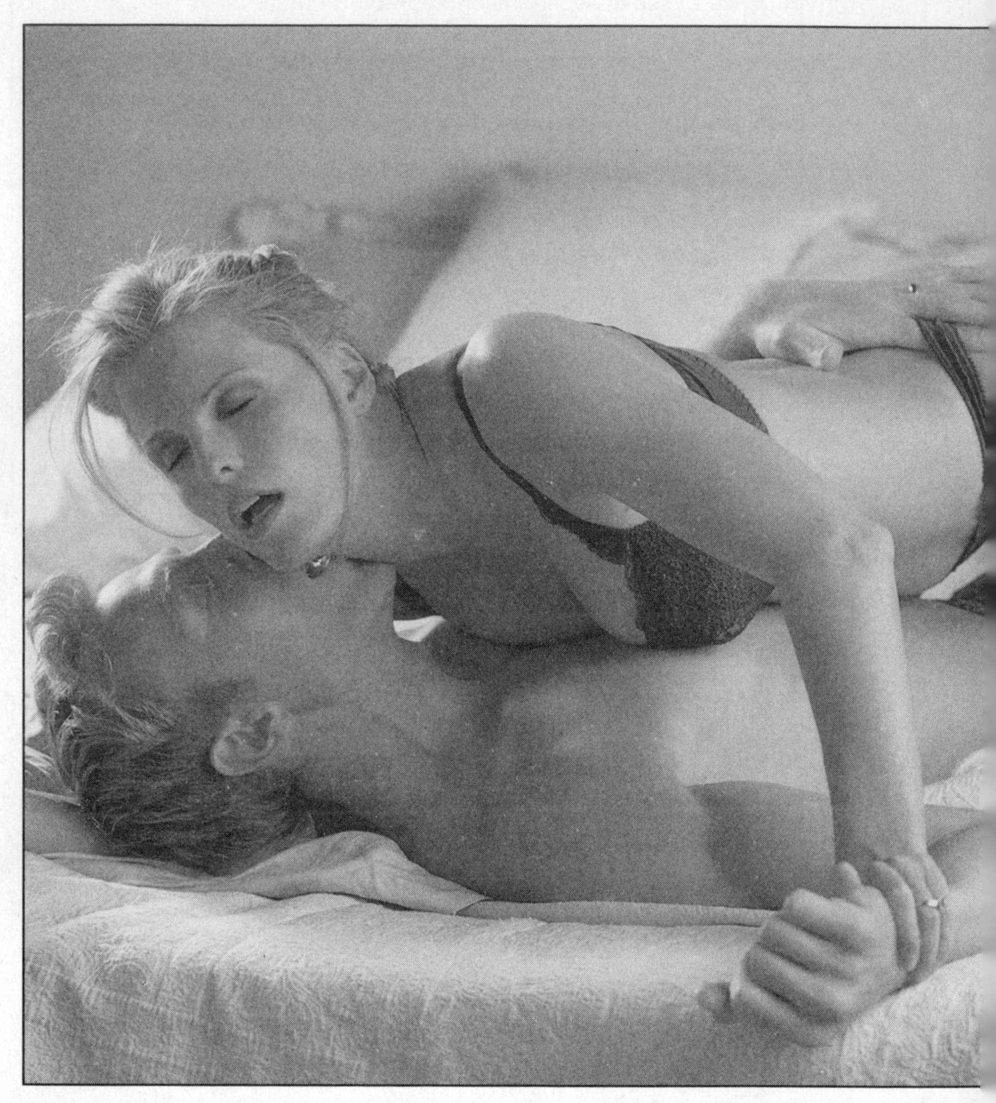

SECRET #6

Multiply Your Pleasure with Multiple and "G-spot" Orgasms

> *Electric flesh-arrows . . . traversing the body. A rainbow of color strikes the eyelids. A foam of music falls over the ears. It is the gong of the orgasm.*
>
> —ANAIS NIN
> *Diary of Anais Nin, Vol. 2*

Human sexuality offers all sorts of pleasures, perhaps few as fulfilling as the "G-spot" and the multiple orgasm. While the first is reserved for women, men can have multiple orgasms, too. With a lot of practice, you and your partner may learn to enjoy multiple orgasms together during a long, luxurious lovemaking session.

"G" MARKS THE SPOT

Ancient erotic texts suggest that humans have known about the "G-spot" for thousands of years. In modern times, though, this pleasure zone has been the source of much debate. In other words, the folks who study sexuality as a science don't all agree on its function. But that has done nothing to dissuade the many women who are true believers in the primacy of the "G-spot" in providing a woman with sexual fulfillment. They firmly believe that learning to locate and pleasure the "G-spot" opens up a whole new level of sensual satisfaction.

The "G-spot," named for a mid nineteenth century German gynecologist named Ernst Grafenberg who identified this erogenous zone, is located within the front (anterior) vaginal wall a few inches inside the vaginal opening—about halfway between the pubic bone and the front of the cervix. The location can vary by several inches from woman to woman. While a male partner can help a woman find her "G-spot," it's very useful for the woman to find it on her own. Here are some instructions:

Women: How to Find Your "G-spot"

This will be a lot more pleasurable if you spend some time getting yourself in a sensual mood. Take a nice, warm bubble bath to relax. Put on some sexy music. Light a candle in your bedroom. Slip into something comfortable that makes you feel luscious. (Just make sure it doesn't constrict your legs.) You may even want to stimulate some of your erogenous zones or bring yourself to clitoral orgasm first.

The reason for all this foreplay is that for some women the "G-spot" swells and hardens when they're aroused. Not only does this swelling make finding the "G-spot" easier, it makes the discovery so much more enjoyable.

Once you've prepared, squat down. This may be easier than reclining. The "G-spot" is almost impossible to find if you're reclining. Insert two lubricated fingers into your vagina and slide them up and down the front vaginal wall (the one closest to your belly button). If you notice a dime-to-half-dollar-sized raised area about a few inches up the wall that feels different than the surrounding area—a little spongier and slightly ridged—you've found your "G-spot."

Don't be discouraged if you don't feel anything. Some women's "G-spots" appear higher in their vaginas. Other women's "G-spots" are less like spots than areas, causing them to feel a more general sensitivity along the front vaginal wall. And many women's fingers simply aren't long enough to reach their "G-spots." A curved vibrator (see Chapter 7) or your partner's fingers may be better suited for that.

Once you've located your pleasure spot, apply a firm, upward pressure, curling your fingers in a "come hither" motion. Experiment with tickles, circles, presses and taps for several minutes. Different strokes delight different folks when it comes to the "G-spot," and some women even prefer different strokes on different occasions.

How do you know when you're on the money? At first, you may feel a sudden urge to urinate. (Although this feeling usually passes, some women like to empty their bladders before "G-spot" play due to its proximity to the urethra.) Many women also report feeling a pleasurable "bearing-down" sensation when they apply pressure to their "G-spots." Women in the throes of "G-spot" ecstasy describe the sensation as "deeply arousing" or "an intense humming sensation" that's just as pleasant, but more diffuse out over the whole body than clitoral sensation.

Question: I've tried stimulating my "G-spot" by myself and with my partner for over a year now. But I still don't feel anything special. Is there something wrong with me?

Not every woman enjoys "G-spot" stimulation. Fortunately, your body offers plenty of other erogenous zones to choose from for sexual activity. Honor your body's unique set of preferences and responses.

If your "G-spot" doesn't seem to be responding— or even feels irritated by the attention—give it some time. "G-spot" stimulation may feel only mildly pleasant or even uncomfortable at first. Realize, too, that not every woman experiences "G-spot" sensitivity. Commit to giving it attention over the next few months, so you can see if the sensation changes. That will let you know whether "G-spot" stimulation is right for you.

"G-spot" Stimulation as a Partner Activity

Once a woman has found her "G-spot," she might want to show her partner how to find it and how she likes to have it pleasured. Since "G-spot" stimulation is such an intense and intimate activity, it's a good idea to start with foreplay rather than diving right in. The longer you spend warming up—whispering sweet nothings, teasing nipples, stroking the vulva, and even engaging in intercourse—the greater your potential for "G-spot" pleasure. And the more "G-spot" pleasure, the better everything else about sex can feel.

It might be easiest for the woman to help her man find her "G-spot" if she gets down on her hands and knees, lowers her head and tilts her pelvis slightly upward. If that's not comfortable, the woman may want to lie on her back and place a large pillow beneath her bottom so that it helps tilt the pelvis. Then her partner can slide two lubricated fingers into her vagina (palm downward if the woman is on her knees, palm upward if she's on her back) and probe the front wall of the vagina. Women, let your man know what feels good. Tilt and rotate your pelvis into his hand to guide him.

The man can increase sensation by using his free hand to press downward on the woman's abdomen, just above the pubic hairline.

As you may recall, Chapter 5 discussed the positions best capable of stimulating the "G-spot" during intercourse. You may want to review that, experiment some, and see which intercourse postures provide the best "G-spot" stimulation. Many women find that shorter (rather than deep) stokes during intercourse work best here. Slight changes in angle or direction of motion can also enhance "G-spot" participation. Women who've experienced them say "G-spot" orgasms feel "less centralized," "deeper," and "more internal" than clitoral climaxes.

With the proper stimulation, some women can experience both "G-spot" and clitoral orgasms at the same time. The woman may want to try using one hand to stimulate the clitoris while the other attends to the "G-spot," or using one hand on the "G-spot" while her partner tongues her clitoris, or holding a vibrator to her clitoris during intercourse. Women who've experienced this report that these orgasms are extremely satisfying.

For Women: Exercising Your "G-spot"

Many believe that "G-spot" sensitivity is directly related to the strength of a woman's pubococcygeus, or PC, muscle. The PC is a group of muscles that run from the pubic bone to the tailbone, creating a sling that supports the internal organs in both women and men. The nerves in this muscle group may also help carry sensation signals from the sex organs to the brain.

To strengthen your PC, try a specially designed workout called Kegels. Named after gynecologist Dr. Arnold Kegel, this exercise was developed during the 1940s to help women control problems with urinary incontinence. Many of the women who originally practiced Kegels for bladder control noticed an amazing side benefit—enhanced sexual pleasure. Some experienced orgasms for the first time, while other participants started enjoying more powerful orgasms, greater "G-spot" arousal, and even multiple orgasms.

These days, doctors often recommend Kegels for women after childbirth to tone loose PC muscles. But there's no need to wait until you've had a baby. Kegels can help almost any woman enhance her PC muscle tone.

To isolate the PC muscle, next time you go to the bathroom, try stopping your flow of urine in midstream. That muscle you're squeezing is the PC muscle. Once you've identified the PC muscle and isolated it, so that you are squeezing it alone, and not the muscles in your stomach and buttocks, you can do Kegels anywhere. Practice squeezing and relaxing your PC in equal three-second intervals. (Don't skimp on the relaxation half of the exercise—it's just as important as the squeezing.) Start with ten repetitions, three times a day, then gradually build up duration and reps. (If this proves too strenuous, just do as many Kegels as you can and build up your strength from there.) The important thing is keeping a regular routine—without overdoing them.

You may not even have to wait to experience Kegel's sensual benefits. Some people report getting aroused while doing the exercise, as well as experiencing more powerful orgasms during later sexual encounters.

Tip: *Women may get even better results from their PC exercises by using vaginal barbells. These smooth little steel sexual aids are shaped like miniature barbells. You insert one into your vagina just before doing Kegels. The additional weight the device supplies not only helps build the PC muscle, it also provides something pleasurable to squeeze against.*

"G-spot" Expulsion

Some women occasionally expel an odorless, clear or milky fluid through the urethral opening in the vulva during "G-spot" stimulation. The amount varies from woman to woman, and from one time to the next— it may be a slight trickle or a veritable gush of fluid. Expulsion may be unrelated to orgasm or it might directly precede it. Many women who experience this before orgasm say it makes the orgasm feel even more satisfying than usual. Others say it's an interesting but neutral experience in terms of orgasm and pleasure. Some women who've learned to expel fluids are quite proud of the feat and like to show off their capabilities. Other women may find the expulsion embarrassing, perhaps fearing that they've accidentally urinated while in the throes of passion.

While you may never learn to beam with pride, research indicates that this fluid is not urine (although it may contain small traces). Rather, it's a substance similar in characteristic to the male prostate fluid that is released along with sperm in male ejaculate. It's perfectly okay for women to experience this, and perfectly okay if they don't.

Women who want to experience this should keep doing their Kegels and stimulating their "G-spot" so they grow more and more aroused by the practice. The more swelling in the "G-spot" from arousal, the more likely that the women will experience orgasm and expel fluid. But it's no guarantee. Even a woman who is extremely aroused and experiences a powerful orgasm might not expel fluid. Some women can develop the ability to expel fluid through practice, but not all women. In any event, it shouldn't be set as a goal.

Multiple Orgasms for Women

Many women turn a skeptical eye toward the phenomenon of multiple orgasms— a series of climaxes with little or no rest in between the peaks. After all, how is it possible to have ten orgasms during a single sexual encounter when achieving one takes so much time, effort, and energy?

The multiple orgasms issue resolves itself differently for each woman. Some will experience them, some will not; some will love them while others will prefer a single orgasm; some will prefer them on some occasions, and a single orgasm on others. As usual, it's up to each individual to establish her own preferences. Women, if you've never experienced multiple orgasms but are interested, you may be able to teach yourself through these techniques. Eventually, most of these practices can be integrated into intercourse. But it will probably be easier to apply them first during masturbation to help your body absorb the extra stimulation and ease into multiple orgasms. Here's what to do:

After masturbating yourself to one orgasm, back off of the intensity of stimulation, but keep touching yourself lightly. Increase the pressure when you're ready. By not quitting stimulation completely after an orgasm, you can keep yourself on an "excitement plateau" from which you can more easily launch into another orgasm.

Try using a vibrator. Many women first experience multiple orgasm with the help of a vibrator. By using a combination of stimulators—hands, vibrators, and dildos—a woman can vary her pleasure and maximize her multi-orgasmic potential. (See Chapter 7 for more information on vibrators and dildos.)

If you prefer, use your fingers. Although the fingers aren't as powerful as a vibrator, they still play an important role for most multi-orgasmic women.

If you're in the habit of masturbating in one particular position, try self-stimulation in several different postures—particularly those in which you most enjoy intercourse.

Breath control may play an important part in having more than one orgasm. Notice how you breathe when you masturbate. Some women hold their breath before they orgasm. See if you can train yourself to continue breathing deeply through your first orgasm and into the next one.

Relax. Focusing on achieving multiple orgasms puts so much pressure on the experience, you may never even arrive at the first one. So relax and just enjoy. Surrender to the sensation and the multiple orgasm may just overtake you. If you take the attitude that you are willing to receive it as a gift, rather than demand it of your body, you may be more likely to experience it.

Experiment with "G-spot" stimulation. Most women rely solely on clitoral stimulation during masturbation. But many multiorgasmic women say that it's easier to have successive "G-spot" orgasms than multiple clitoral climaxes. So be sure to try stimulating the "G-spot" as you explore your capacity for multiple orgasms.

When you've learned to climax several times on your own, you may be able to apply these skills during intercourse. But don't be discouraged if you can't.

Multiple Orgasm for Men

Although many men realize that women can be multiorgasmic, few seem to know that they share that potential. The confusion is understandable, especially since men usually zone out right after they ejaculate. (Ejaculation does exhaust body and mind.) Multiple orgasm is possible because male orgasm and ejaculation are separate physiological processes. In more concrete terms, that quickening of the heart and warm flush that moves throughout your body— and the fluid that propels itself out the end of your penis—don't need to happen simultaneously. You can learn to experience that body-thrilling rush characteristic of orgasm without emitting semen. This way, you can enjoy several orgasms before ejaculation—and have a better chance of affording your partner the same experience. Ancient texts offer men a number of strategies for achieving this. The technique is described in detail below.

Why would any man want to bother to learn how to separate the process of ejaculation from the process of orgasmic release? Well, men who've had multiple orgasms describe the experience in almost reverent terms. They say multiples sometimes feel "deeper," or "richer," than a single orgasm, and can help them prolong the pleasure of making love. When you forgo ejaculation, you forgo exhaustion so you can make love longer.

Men: How to Orgasm Without Ejaculating

Men, the next step to becoming multiorgasmic is talking yourself into the possibility of it. Close your eyes and imagine having an orgasm. Recall how your whole body feels during the experience. Begin stimulating your penis through masturbation. Concentrate on taking long, deep, belly-expanding breaths while bringing yourself closer to orgasm. By relaxing and focusing on something besides ejaculation, you can attune yourself to all the body processes going on during sexual climax. In addition to an elevated heart rate and warm flush, men experience a number of rhythmic contractions in their genitals during orgasm—just like women do. Become familiar with how these contractions feel, and how many you typically experience during orgasms. Experiment and see how many contractions you can have before ejaculation hits. See if you can have just one or two extra contractions without going over the edge. Gradually, you can learn to relax into the orgasm and experience more and more contractions without ejaculation. Try these methods for extending sexual control and pleasure. Give yourself permission to explore this over the next few weeks.

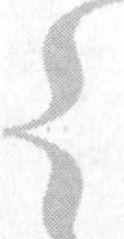

Tip: *Kegels can be just as beneficial for men. Strong PC muscles may help males enhance their orgasms and develop multi-orgasmic capacity.*

Techniques for Ejaculatory Control

Using a lubricant, stimulate your penis to just before the point of ejaculatory inevitability (the moment when you know you're going to ejaculate and nothing you can do will stop it—not even thinking about moving). Stop and breathe deeply, slowing down or stopping stimulation whenever you feel that you're approaching the edge. You'll probably go right over the edge the first few times you try. But eventually, you will be able to master the process so you can stop yourself at the point just before ejaculation.

Try building up to, and then stopping at, this point as many times as you can over the course of a single masturbation session.

Pleasure other parts of your body during masturbation and focus on them. Stimulate your nipples, stroke your thighs and perineum, fondle your testicles. Relax as much as you can and focus on your entire body. It feels wonderful and provides great training for the sensuality of prolonged lovemaking.

Try applying firm, rhythmic pressure on the prostate gland. this will duplicate the contractions of first-stage orgasm without stimulating the ejaculatory reflex. (See Chapter 10 for more information.) Some have coined this the "P-spot," for convenience, although it does not refer to an actual anatomical site, like the "G-spot."

The Multiple Couple

Extended lovemaking, in ways that allow both of you to reach multiple orgasm, can bring extraordinary pleasure. But don't expect perfection at first. In fact, using these techniques might feel clumsy at first. So have a sense of humor about it and don't get too caught up in counting orgasms or reaching your goal. Couples who are successful with extended lovemaking focus on the pleasure of the experience, and let the orgasms happen in their own time.

Here are some tips that can help:

- Get the whole body involved. Put less emphasis on genital stimulation— especially the man's— and expand the pleasure to the entire body. Moving from the penis to a different body part just before ejaculation is a great way for women to keep their partners on a high pleasure plateau without sending them over the edge. Most people enjoy having their lover pleasure the entire body, which feels more luxurious than concentrating all the sensations just on the genitals.

• Don't let opposites detract. Keep in mind, that men and women employ essentially contradictory techniques to achieve extended sexual arousal. Men reduce stimulation at key moments to avoid ejaculation, while women usually need to increase stimulation or use different kinds of touching to climax again and again.

• Communication is as essential as ever. Women need to educate their men on what feels best. And men need to let women know what feels good too, especially when they're approaching ejaculation.

• Take a break. If the man pauses during intercourse to pleasure the woman manually and/or orally, he can increase her level of excitement while allowing him to pace himself so he can keep going.

• The Tease. Couples can practice extending their pleasure to exquisite lengths by varying their touch and alternating light stimulation with intense thrusting, always stopping before either partner goes over the edge.

If you'd like to see a visual presentation of the material in this chapter, refer to the following video from the Sinclair Intimacy Institute Video Library: Volume 2 of The Better Sex Video Series®: *Unlocking the Secrets of the G-Spot.*

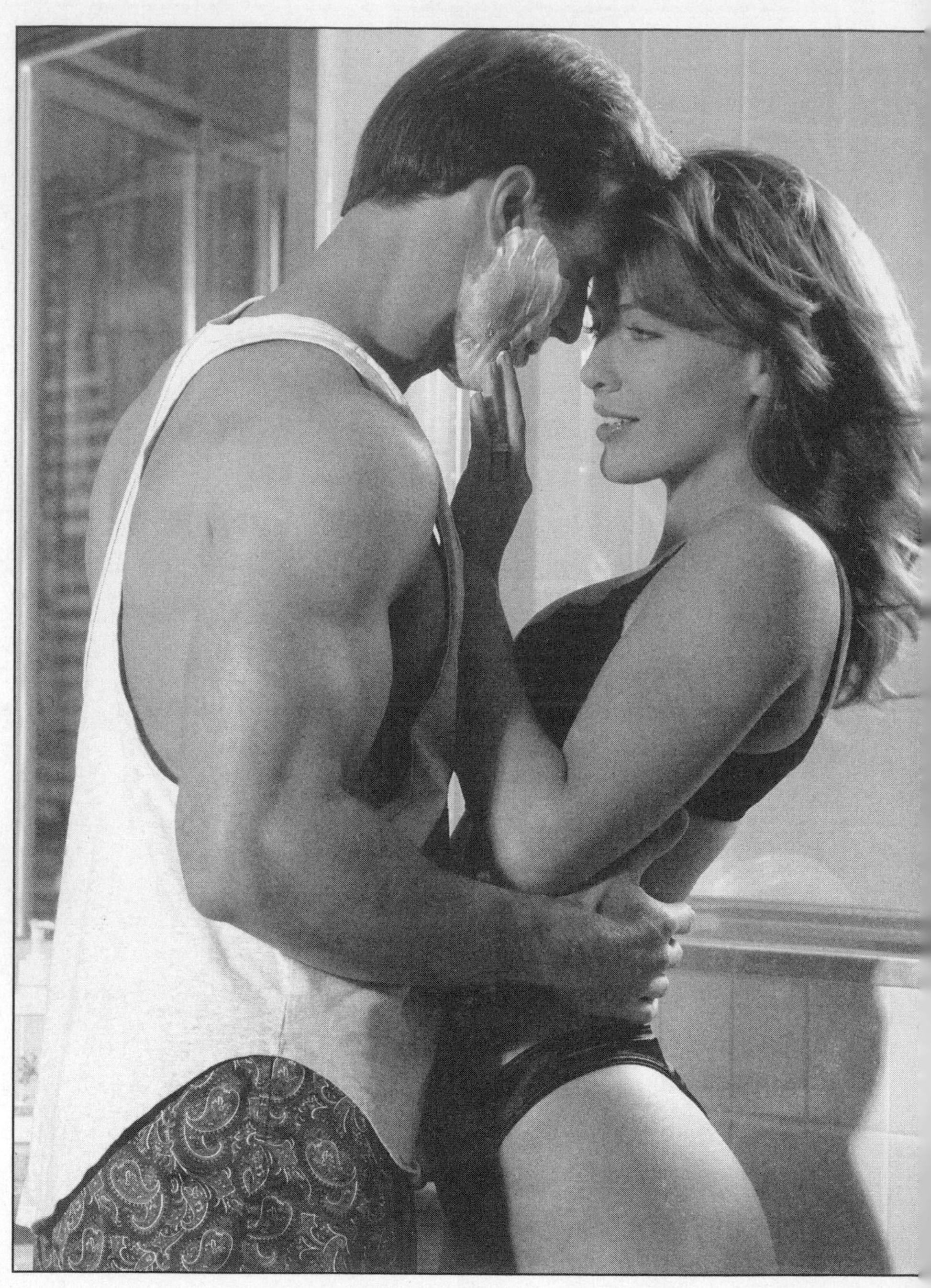

SECRET #7

Make Sex Fun With Toys

That was the most fun I've ever had without laughing.

—WOODY ALLEN
Annie Hall

Think of sex as playtime for adults. Let it engage your imagination, creativity and sense of humor. Certainly, you can bring all of these to your intimate encounters without ever using an adult video, an erotic game, a vibrator, or a cock ring. If that's not your style, skip to the next chapter. But if you are curious about how couples can use these products to heighten their sexual satisfaction, read on.

BORED? TRY BOARD AND OTHER GAMES

If your sexual routine is a little tired, consider perking it up with a fun game designed to enhance intimacy. There are a number of good ones on the market. These can help you bring more playfulness to your intimate time together. "The More Foreplay Game," for instance, uses spinners to encourage couples to explore thousands of different erotic possibilities. Some games can even help you and your partner dissolve barriers to intimacy, because they ask questions that get at your deepest desires. The "Speak Love, Make Love Game," for instance, is a two-sided board game designed to help couples explore their fantasies and desires. "An Enchanted Evening Game" draws players around the board in a fun and enlightening competition to draw up a "Secret Wish" list. As in all sex games, there are no losers, just players. You can find games like these at lingerie or novelty shops, or online markets like Bettersex.com.

Non-sexual adult games can also be adapted for sensual play. Consider how poker became "strip poker" and think of how you can adapt your favorite card games, board games and sporting activities accordingly. Consider, too, how many of the best couple's games happen spontaneously—the silly tickle and giggle sessions in bed, the impromptu dance maneuvers, the bubble-blowing and hoola-hoop sessions you might get into while cleaning up the kids' toys. These playful moments create much of the fabric of your love.

Playing Together with Sex Toys

Sex toys and accessories can also add a new dimension, as well as new sensations, to your intimate time together. If you haven't explored these, don't automatically think "whips and chains." There are tamer products, as well as some you might consider over the top.

On the tamer side are tasteful couple's videos, such as our instructional sex education videos, or other erotic videos that feature couples in loving relationships. You might find that the right ones heat you both up and teach you new "tricks" you can add to your repertoire of lovemaking skills. Vibrators can be used as part of foreplay to pleasure each other, or even as an aid in sensual massage. Tickler sleeves can add pleasure in intercourse. Constriction rings, also known as cock rings, can help men maintain erections. Men can also use accessories called male masturbators—usually molded to look like a vagina or jellyroll, and filled with a soft, slippery surface. Some even simulate the "sucking" sensation a man might experience during fellatio. These can be useful in sex play when a man engages in self-pleasuring to attain a firm enough erection for intercourse.

There are even more exotic accessories, like anal beads, anal vibrators, or "anal training kits" designed for use by those who enjoy anal intercourse or want to experiment with it. There are also sexual toys such as whips and restraints, as well as more unusual accessories like "cock locks," for the those who are into sadism and masochism, or dominance and submission.

It can be a lot of fun to sit down with your partner and look through a catalogue full of sex toys and talk about what you want. If you choose not to keep such catalogues around the house because you're concerned your children might find them, you can also find catalogues on the Web at sites such as Bettersex.com, which is the web store of The Sinclair Intimacy Institute. Of course, you can also find some of these products locally, in a lingerie store or an adult pleasure emporium, but you might find that you prefer talking about what you want in the privacy of your own home, even before you venture out to do the actual shopping. Speaking of shopping, you'll want to be as choosy here as you are when you make any other type of purchase. Try to stick with reputable companies and catalogues. The sex toys on the market vary in quality.

To aid you in your discussion, here's a rundown on different kinds of toys and accessories that may enhance your sexual play:

The Buzz on Vibrators

Sensual vibrating devices were used by the medical profession as early as the late nineteenth century to treat what they referred to as "female hysteria." The doctors were bringing their female patients to orgasm in their offices, and women kept returning for "treatments." Today, vibrators are designed for individuals, and are strictly a "pleasure" purchase. They come in a wide range of styles and sizes, and provide different forms of stimulation. External vibrators are used to stimulate the clitoris and other sensitive areas of the vulva. They are great at providing enough stimulation to bring a woman to orgasm. They can also be used, perhaps on a lower setting, to pleasure a man's testicles, and penis. Couples who've never tried an external vibrator might find it fun to introduce it into their sex play by using it as a massager. Let yourself feel how the vibration stimulates your neck, back and arms before you move it to more sensitive areas.

External vibrators come in a variety of models. Electric coil vibrators funnel strong, high-frequency vibrations to a relatively concentrated area. They serve as a great basic sex toy for those who appreciate a strong, semi-silent vibrator that does the job. Some coil vibrators come with multiple attachments: one for the woman, one for the man, one for internal use, and one for external use.

Wand vibrators diffuse vibrations over a larger area. Many women who have difficulty reaching orgasm achieve their first orgasms with the soft ball-shaped head of this toy. Like the coil vibrator, the wand vibrator can be used with attachments. Some couples also enjoy using the wand for clitoral stimulation during intercourse. This can be pleasurable for both partners, as men may feel the vibrations of this powerful tool through their partner's genitals.

Shopping for Toys

When you two are ready to go on your first "sexpedition" together, consider looking for a store that bills itself as "sex positive." Stores like Good Vibrations in San Francisco, for instance, have a pleasant atmosphere and very informed salespeople. These stores are not sleazy, unlike the triple X type shop you often see in the seedier parts of town.

Buying from a store offers a few benefits over mail-order shopping. You can actually see and feel what you're going to buy. You might learn something new from looking at the merchandise or talking to the staff. And it can be a fun, stimulating experience for you and your partner.

A decent store shouldn't be difficult for you to find. See if your local lingerie shop carries a selection of sex toys. (You may be more successful if you look for a "mom and pop" run business that's outside the local mall.) If you can't find what you want locally, however, there are always mail-order catalogues and electronic ones on the Web. Most companies package merchandise discretely, so you don't have to worry about the postman spreading gossip.

If you're not sure what amount of stimulation you like, or your preference for different levels tends to vary, look for multi-speed vibrators. These units allow you to set different vibrational intensity levels, to fit your mood and circumstances.

If you are concerned about privacy because you're sharing a home with children, a parent or other relative, look for a quiet vibrator. The sound of some vibrators is unmistakable. You don't want to tense up every time you turn on the vibrator because you're afraid someone will hear it.

Another variable to consider is the power source. Electric-powered vibrators tend to be stronger and longer lasting, but some people prefer the gentler vibrations of battery-operated toys. Battery units also don't require an electrical outlet, so they're much more portable. Some battery-operated vibrators even come with a remote control unit. The vibrator part is typically tucked into a special panty. That lets the partner work the remote control, giving him or her the ability to turn it on and off from distances of up to five yards. Think of the fun the two of you can have, fooling around with something like that. Realize, however, that most remote-powered vibrators make quite a bit of noise. That might be okay in a noisy nightclub, but you might not want to use it in a quiet French restaurant unless you and your partner are real exhibitionists.

There are also vibrators that attach to the hand, and turn fingers into little pleasure machines. Many couples also enjoy using these during foreplay and intercourse. Fingertip devices allow you to fine-tune the pressure and location of vibrations. They also offer superior mobility, allowing for the stimulation of different erogenous zones in quick succession.

Although external units offer unbeatable clitoral stimulation, many women also enjoy the vaginal pressure and sensation they can only get from insertable vibrators, designed for insertion into the vagina. Insertable vibrators come in many different styles. Some are "realistic," or penis-shaped. These do a particularly good job of stimulating the sensitive nerves at the opening of the vagina. But some women, who still aren't comfortable with the idea of using a sex toy, prefer other shapes, such as egg-shaped vibrators or those that are smooth and cylindrical. There are even insertable vibrators that are angled for "G-spot" stimulation.

> **Tip:** *You can use a condom on insertable sex toys so that they stay clean and don't transmit germs into your body. Or clean the toys after each use with a disinfectant such as hydrogen peroxide. Internal sex toys can transmit bacteria and diseases so it's not a good idea to share one with a partner without using these precautions.*

Insertable vibrators are battery-operated. They tend to be made of rubber, plastic, vinyl and latex. If you're purchasing from a store, take it out of the box, and feel the surface of the vibrator to determine which you like the best. Make sure you're not allergic to a particular material. (Those with latex sensitivities should choose other options when it comes to sex toys and products.)

Many women prefer insertable vibrators made of pliable materials rather than hard plastic. Others like the plastic because of the fun colors and patterns. Whichever you choose, consider picking up a bottle of water-based lubricant when you buy your vibrator. That may make vibrator play even more enjoyable. If you like anal play, you might also want to pick up a package of lubricated condoms, so you can sheath the vibrator with a new condom each time you use it. This way, you prevent importing bacteria from the anus into the vagina and vice versa.

Some couples like dual-purpose vibrators, especially during foreplay. These have an internal vibrator that stimulates the vagina, plus as an external one that stimulates the clitoris. (The external vibrator, designed to flutter over the clitoris, sometimes features a "cute" animal shape, like a dolphin.) The internal vibrating shaft may swivel, or employ other kinds of sensual movement, to stimulate the sensitive vaginal nerves. Dual-purpose vibrators don't always replace a basic external vibrator when it comes to effective clitoral stimulation. But they can be an extremely pleasurable addition to your sex-toy chest.

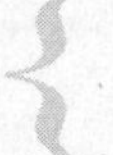

Tip: *To lessen the intensity of a vibrator, try using it with a silk scarf or a thin piece of clothing between you and the toy.*

Men and Vibrators

Guys, don't think vibrators are just for women. They can also be used on male erogenous zones. Just be sure to choose vibrators with low settings so that the vibration isn't too intense to be pleasurable. Here are just a few of the possibilities:

- Try using a cup attachment on a basic coil vibrator to stimulate the head of the penis.

- Run a wand vibrator up and down the shaft of the penis.

- Hold a fingertip vibrator on the sensitive strip of skin behind the testicles (the perineum) to add sensation during manual or oral stimulation.

- Use a vibrator to stimulate the nipples.

Question: I just got my first vibrator and it's terrific. But I'm afraid my husband may get a little jealous. How do I introduce my new toy to him?

It sounds like you're afraid your partner may be a little threatened by your mechanical friend. This is a very common concern. After all, no human lover could stimulate you at the 2000 vibrations per minute that many vibrators are capable of. Vibrators can be so good they're intimidating. Many therapists recommend that couples buy a sex toy together. But since you've gone ahead and taken the initiative, you'll need to go to plan B: a thoughtful, polite introduction.

When introducing your sex toy to your lover, try to use a direct but very sensitive approach. Assure him that a machine could never replace his special, human touch. Tell him (or better yet, show him) that using a vibrator doesn't use up your desire but increases it. Invite him to use the vibrator with you by stimulating your body as you use the toy, and by massaging him with it.

If he's game, let him try it on his genitals while you stimulate his other erogenous zones. There's nothing like pleasure to create a positive impression. By the time you're finished introducing your new sex toy to your mate, he may even want a mechanical friend of his own.

Another "toy" designed for male pleasure is the male masturbator mentioned above. These come in many models, and attempt to simulate the feel of the vagina. These are terrific for husbands whose jobs take them on the road a lot, giving them an alternative to manual masturbation when it isn't possible for them to engage in sex play with their wives. Research shows that men who remain sexually active are less likely to get prostate cancer.

Dildos: Always Ready For Action

Dildos, perhaps the most ancient of sex toys, mimic the penis in form and function. Certainly, they don't have the warmth or special loving energy of a penis. But they are always ready for action. These come in a wide variety of shapes, colors, textures and sizes. Most are meant to be hand-held, but a few are designed to fit into a harness, which a partner can wear. Here's a brief review of features you'll want to consider if you're thinking about purchasing one:

SHAPE

Some women enjoy the look and feel of "realistic" dildos that have ridges and veins similar to those of a penis. Other women prefer smooth, cylindrical dildos. Still others swear by ones that curve backward to pleasure the "G-spot." You may want to try all three.

TEXTURE

Dildos come in plastic and rubber and other synthetic materials. Many experts recommend silicone dildos. Although they're a little more expensive than those made of other materials, they're smooth, firm but pliable, and warm up nicely. And because silicone is nonporous and easier to clean than dildos made of other materials, it's more hygienic.

COLOR

Dildos come in every color of the rainbow and then some. If you like shocking pink, you can have it. If you want leopard skin, you can have that, too. Don't forget to make attractiveness a consideration, too.

INTERCOURSE AIDS

Constriction rings, typically called cock rings, are straps or bands that fit around the testicle and shaft of the penis and keep blood from flowing out of the penis. They can help men maintain erections that may be slightly harder, larger and even more pleasurable than normal. (However, they are not meant to compensate for erectile dysfunction.)

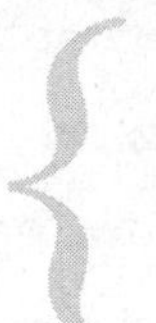

Tip: *Men with certain medical conditions such as diabetes, vascular and blood clotting disorders, and those who bleed easily or who are on blood-thinning medications should avoid cock rings and other sex toys that manipulate blood flow.*

Many men (and women) enjoy the way they feel during intercourse. By stretching out the skin, they also make the penis more sensitive. Older men, especially, appreciate cock/constriction rings because they can help prolong erection. Just be aware that cock rings can cause damage if worn too long, so limit your ring-time to 20-30 minutes. By all means, take it off sooner if it feels uncomfortable.

There are several different kinds of cock rings on the market. Some come with little vibrators attached, which stimulate the clitoris, making them a great couple's toy. If you've never tried a cock ring before, read the instructions carefully. You may want to start with one that features a single strap that's adjustable, or is made from a stretchy material that's easy to remove. Getting a cock ring off can be tricky, so become thoroughly familiar with it before getting serious.

For Those of You Who Like to Watch

If you've grown up thinking of adult entertainment as "pornography," you might never consider the idea of watching an erotic video with your partner. But there's reason to reconsider. Contrary to what you might think, not all of them are demeaning to women. Certainly, some are. But there are others that are tasteful and couples-oriented, meaning they tend to have a more romantic story line, men and women who obviously care about each other, and male actors who are as attractive as the actresses. These videos may be pure erotica, or they may be instructional in nature, like the sexual education videos in the Sinclair Video Library.

Watching erotic videos together can be as educational as it is stimulating. You may find that it adds excitement and new skills to your sex play. Most people learn best when they see something demonstrated, and erotic videos provide a front-row seat to sexual encounters you would not otherwise get to see. According to a study conducted by Northeast Louisiana University professor Lamar Woodham. Ed.D. and sex therapist Constance Engel, M.S.W., couples who watch explicit instructional videotapes experience greater satisfaction in their relationships as well as in their sex lives. Eighty-four percent of the women and 82 percent of the men in a study group that watched The Better Sex Video Series® and The Erotic Guide to Sexual Fantasies for Lovers reported experiencing increased pleasure in foreplay, intercourse and oral sex.

Sex videos tend to fall into one of three basic categories: clinical, instructional and entertainment. While some couples may enjoy one type of video more than another, there may be a place for all three in your relationship.

- Clinical videos like Sinclair's *A Man's Guide to Stronger Erections*, *You Can Last Longer: Solutions for Ejaculatory Control* and *Becoming Orgasmic*, deal with specialized issues from a treatment perspective. Although sexually explicit, their focus is on providing clinical information.

- Instructional videos, designed to educate, offer a blend of entertainment and knowledge. They cover every imaginable topic, including creative sexual positions, oral sex and fantasy. They're a great resource for couples looking to learn a few tips, revamp or spice up their sex lives, or for those looking to get back to basics.

• Entertainment videos, which range from the raunchy to the sublime, are designed to titillate. They may create a lot of excitement for you and your partner. Many couples enjoy watching entertainment videos as a form of foreplay. These videos may introduce you to new positions, or inspire you to create the kind of scenarios or role-playing games that fulfill your fantasies. Or the video may satisfy certain fantasies entirely. With these kinds of videos, you want to take care to choose those that offer "sex-positive" messages, depict men and women with respect, and that don't conflict with your values. Finding ones that you and your partner feel good about watching may require discussion and, perhaps, a willingness to compromise.

Tip: *If an erotic video makes you uncomfortable or turns you off, don't hesitate to turn it off. If you feel neutral about it, however, you may want to keep watching it. Even if you don't totally love the look or content of an entire video, there's often a little something that you can take out of it—an interesting new position, an idea for erotic role-playing, or a great erotic toy that you can find and add to your repertoire.*

Keep in mind that most "adult" videos don't have the sophisticated production values of the big-budget movies that you are used to watching. So you'll either have to lower your aesthetic standards or search long and hard for "porn" that features good cinematography, interesting story lines, and handsome men as well as attractive women.

Before you make the effort to find videos you'll enjoy, set time aside to talk to each other about what you want. Each of you should be honest with the other about what would turn you on, what would turn

Make Your Own Erotic Video

Videotaping each other in various states of sex play can be an erotic adventure. Almost everyone has a little voyeur or exhibitionist deep down inside them, and home video production offers a fun way to tap into that erotic energy.

A few ideas for playing director with your partner:

- Dim the lights, use candles, or try a colored light bulb to create a flattering ambiance.
- Think like a photographer and "dress" your partner's naked body with sexy shadows like the stripes of venetian blinds or the patterns of window lace as they reflect on the bed.
- If your lover feels self-conscious, have them choose a fun costume or sexy disguise so they can get "in character."
- Concentrate on angles that play up your partner's favorite body parts. Even professional actors and actresses need to be shot from flattering angles in order to look sexy.

Videotaping each other can make for great sex play, but it's no fun to get caught. Don't forget to erase the tape or hide it in an ultra secure place when you're done. You don't want a friend, housekeeper or child coming across it and popping it into the VCR. If you just want to enjoy the act of videotaping without the worry, don't press the record button.

you off, what fears you might have about watching such videos and what you absolutely will not watch and do not want in your home. You may learn a lot about each other in the process.

Once the two of you know what you're looking for, the fun begins. Just be aware that it may take a lot of trial and error to find videos that work for both of you. A good way to find couple-friendly videos is to look to your favorite web site for guidance. Some sites include ratings that specifically designate videos as "woman-centered," "good plot," or "couples-oriented." After you've watched several of these videos and determined a style you like, look to see who directed your favorite video. Then see if you can find more by that director. Some directors who focus on making couples-oriented videos are Candida Royalle, Paul Thomas and Andrew Blake.

If you'd like to see a visual presentation of the material in this chapter, refer to the following videos from the Sinclair Intimacy Institute Video Library: Volume 3 of The Better Sex Video Series®: *Making Sex Fun,* and *Toys for Better Sex.*

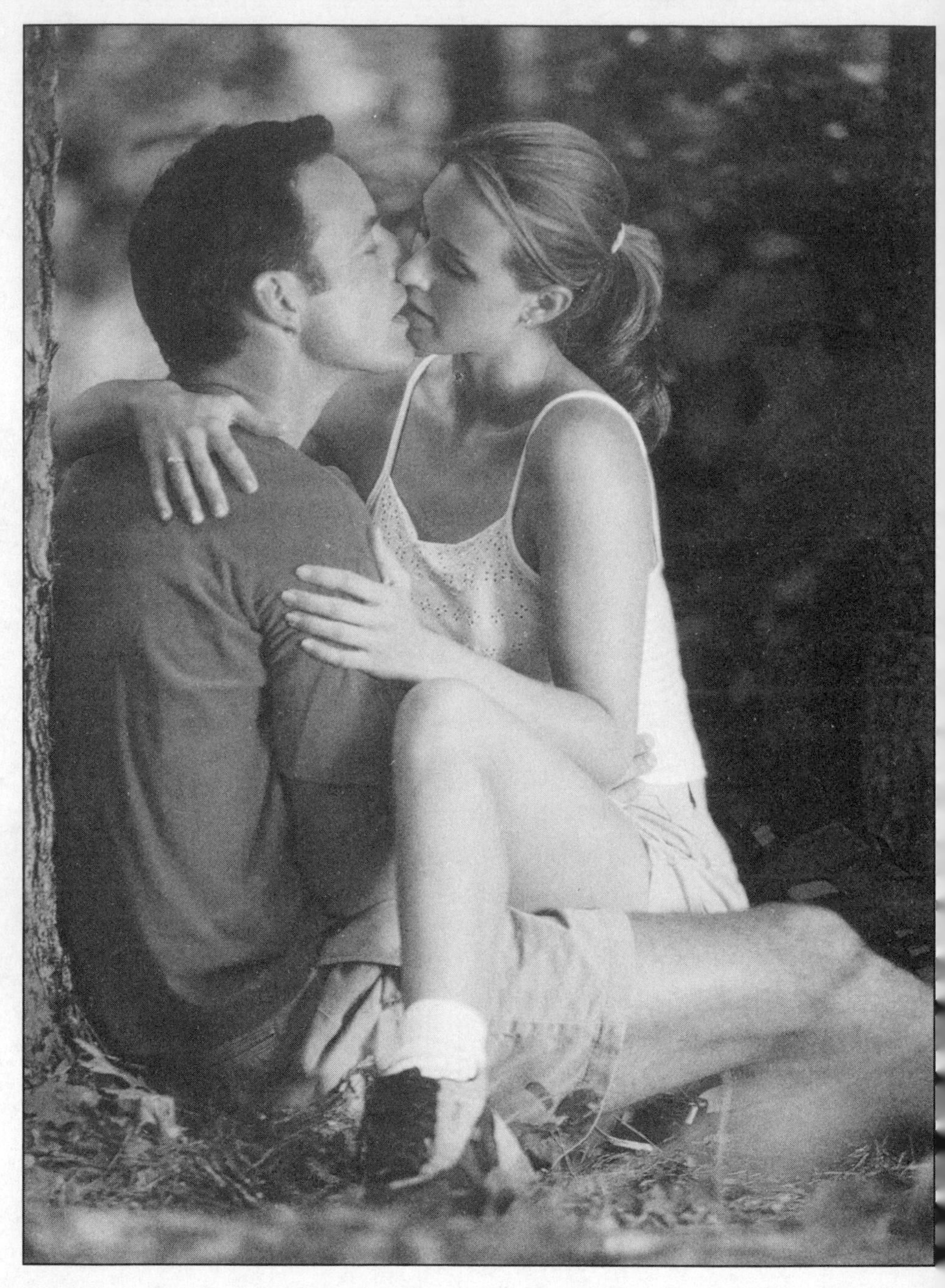

Secret #8

Seek Stimulating Settings

Variety is the soul of pleasure.

—Aphra Behn
The Rover

The human brain seeks variety, and new forms of stimulation. So does the human animal. That's why relegating sex to the bedroom only becomes boring after a while. Finding different places to experience physical intimacy can bring a freshness to your time together. If you haven't talked about this, you might want to set aside some time to brainstorm about other places where the two of you could make love. You may even discover that you and your partner share a similar longing for a tryst at a secluded beach at sunset, or in the waterfall pool of a mountain stream. Or maybe what you really want is time in one of those cheesy rent-by-the-hour motel rooms where you can make as much noise as you want, without worrying about being overhead by your children, or that nosy elderly neighbor next door. If cash is tight, and your car or minivan has a roomy enough backseat, you could even "park," just as you did when you were a teenager. You may want to stick to the garage, a secluded driveway or someplace just as safe, so you don't put yourselves in danger.

If travel money is tight, also consider exploring what your region has to offer in terms of romantic bed-and-breakfasts and/or campgrounds. Of course, you don't have to ever leave your front door to experience alternatives to "bedroom sex." Consider surprising your partner with an erotic embrace in one of the following rooms:

- **The Kitchen.** Counters, tables and chairs can take sex to literally new heights as you experience intimate contact at different elevations and angles. The kitchen is also a terrific place to seduce your partner by rubbing ice cubes on each other's lips and neck, or applying dessert to your naked body. If you've got the house to yourselves, there's no need to head to the bedroom once you've seduced each other.

- **The Bathroom.** Many couples find aquatic sex play absolutely wonderful. If you don't have a hot tub or private pool, play together in your shower or tub. See how much fun you can have with bubble baths, sponge massages, detachable showerheads and vibrators designed for water play.

- **Stairways.** Stopping on the stairs for sex seems to scream, "I want you so much I can't wait until we get to the next floor!" Stairs also offer some interesting new angles. Just be sure you're both on stable footing, and keep a grip on the handrail, if it's secure enough to support the extra weight.

• **The Living Room.** If you're lucky enough to have a fireplace with ample room in front of it, or you've decorated with a lot of mirrors, there may be no better place in the house to make love. Even without the fireplace or mirrors, the couch may be way cool for a necking and petting session, especially if you choose to begin your intimate time together by watching an erotic video.

• **The Laundry Room.** The washer and dryer provide sturdy surfaces at or near groin level. If they're in operation, you'll also get some noise cover and interesting vibrations.

• **The Garage or Basement.** These may not offer the comfort of other locations around the house, but it might be interesting to hear the sounds of lovemaking echoing off the floor and walls. Secluded driveways also offer a secure place to park if you'd like to try a tryst in the backseat of your car.

• **The Home Gym.** Some couples enjoy exercising before or just after they make love. For some lovers, sweat—believe it or not—is an aphrodisiac. So is that post-workout glow. Exercise mats, incline benches and crunch boards also offer some interesting possibilities for lovemaking. Just make sure heavy objects like weight bars and barbells are stabilized before starting.

Enhancing the Pleasure Quotient of Your Bedroom

If your living arrangements preclude you from making love anywhere else but behind the locked doors of your bedroom, you can still add some spice. Try surprising your lover by transforming yours. You can go romantic, by adding fresh flowers, scented candles, and soft lighting, or you can decorate it to play out a fantasy, temporarily transforming it into a tropical paradise with water fountains and flowering orchids; an Arabian pleasure palace complete with tent; even a medieval confessional booth, with a wooden "kneeler" and frankincense incense.

Here are some other suggestions:

- Spread some pillows and blankets in interesting new textures, like velvet or silk, on the floor in front of a fireplace or in the living room.

- Fill the room with scented candles or burn incense.

- Bring the hammock in. Or purchase a Love Swing designed for creative sex play.

- Keep an eye out for novelties that could be used in your erotic play. Consider finding a trunk to fill with your sex "finds."

Mara had had a long, hard day at work. As she stumbled into her apartment, she wasn't sure she'd even have the strength for the romantic getaway weekend that her lover Larry had promised. She was so tired, in fact, she thought for a moment that she'd accidentally entered the wrong apartment. The bedroom looked completely different. But there was her trusty clock radio and Eiffel Tower poster on the wall. It was the same room where she slept every night—the same one she'd trudged out of that very morning. Yet it had been completely transformed.

No longer exhausted, Mara felt a tingling of excitement as she surveyed the room. A bouquet of roses stood on the bed stand. The scent of vanilla wafted from a burning candle on the dresser. Sultry soul music poured out of the clock radio's cassette player. The white light bulb over the bed had been replaced by a pink bulb that basked the room in a sexy new glow. Who had done all this and why?

Her questions were answered as her lover Larry stepped into the room wearing only a bathrobe and a smile. He had transformed the bedroom into a "romantic getaway," and they would spend a glorious weekend there talking, laughing, eating, sleeping and making love.

Erotic Travel

Traveling with your lover—whether to a warm beach or a mountain cabin—often seems to stir the libido. Unfamiliar surroundings can increase your intimacy as you explore something new together. Lovers' fondest memories and most intense periods of bonding often occur during their vacations together. That's because travel often affords plenty of opportunity for fun. If you choose an exotic place like Bali, or a Caribbean island, you might even find that some of that native sensuality rubs off on you. Consider the trip an investment in your romantic future—one that could pay dividends for the rest of your lives together.

Sex Au Natural

The desire to make love outdoors is very common. There is something about being in a beautiful setting, and listening to the sounds of nature, that seems to enhance everything. If the two of you decide you'd like to make love outdoors, you might want to pack a picnic meal, making sure to include your favorite sex accessories. Be sure to bring along those items you usually use, like lubricants, battery-operated vibrators (and the condoms to cover them), even washcloths and skin cleanser to help with the clean-up afterward.

Before you begin, be sure to check the "secluded" area for not-so-obvious routes of access. You might also want to check the ground for poison ivy or any other plants that can spark an allergic reaction.

Sam and Lynn ran a small business from their house. Business was going great—maybe a little too great. Lately, it seemed like life was all work. Order forms on the dining room table, a laptop in the bedroom, a long line of calls on the answering machine in the kitchen—no matter where they went in their home, work responsibilities stared back at them.

Lynn realized that they needed to recharge their sensual batteries—and that they had to get out of their home/office to do it. She knew they didn't have the time or money for a long romantic vacation, so she planned a special surprise—a mini-vacation close to home. Lynn told Sam not to schedule any business after 3 p.m. on Friday. She told him a new client was coming over to discuss a "special project"—one that they'd probably need all weekend to get rolling.

On Friday afternoon, Lynn told Sam that she'd accidentally set up another meeting with a long-time client in the restaurant of the local luxury hotel. She asked him to cover it while she met the new client at home. Sam drove to the hotel. When he arrived in the restaurant, no one was there. He was just about to leave when the waiter handed him a phone. Lynn was on the other end of the line. In a sly, sexy tone, she told Sam there was some urgent business for him to attend to up in Room 806.

When Sam entered the room, he saw Lynn sitting on the bed dressed in a sexy nightgown, holding a pair of champagne glasses. She'd taken the other car to the hotel right after Sam, rented the room and filled it with candles and flowers. Sam and Lynn spent the rest of the afternoon drinking champagne and making love. They ate a nice dinner in the restaurant, then hurried back to the room to make love again. Afterwards, they fell asleep in each other's arms. When they awoke in the morning, they felt closer and happier together than they had in weeks. They even made love one more time before checking out and returning home.

Getting out of their house and away from their work responsibilities gave Sam and Lynn a much-needed chance to relax together. It also gave them some perspective on their lives. They decided to make a commitment to spend relaxing evenings together, and to make it a monthly ritual to enjoy a hotel getaway.

Risky Business

With a little planning, you can also turn routine locations into the setting for erotic encounters. An after-hours visit to your lover's office can turn into some afternoon delight on a desk or executive chair. The building's elevator, stairwells or rooftop may also offer possibilities. If you're the one in charge of the planning for these riskier locations, it's your responsibility to make sure the location is safe, private and secure. If you can secure access by locking a door, terrific. Keep an eye out for security cameras, too, or you might end up on tape. Also, consider how the area conducts sound. Being overheard can prove nearly as embarrassing as having someone walk in on the two of you.

Many people actually get more aroused when making love in situations where they might be seen by someone other than their partner. These folks aren't necessarily "exhibitionists," they're just responding to the added tension and thrill of the situation.

Couples who are turned on by the idea of "getting caught" can test out illicit sex play in smaller ways—like teasing each other under a blanket at an outdoor concert or playing footsy under a restaurant tablecloth. If that revs your motors, you might want to shift into a higher gear. Just remember that it's the idea of getting caught that's hot. Actually getting caught might not be so fun, and may put you in an embarrassing situation that's hard to live down. If you're concerned about the risk to your career or your social standing in the community, come up with a creative alternative.

If you'd like to see a visual presentation of the material in this chapter, refer to the following videos from the Sinclair Intimacy Institute Video Library: Volumes 1 and 3 of The Better Sex Video Series®: *Sexual Positions for Lovers,* and *10 Secrets to Great Sex.*

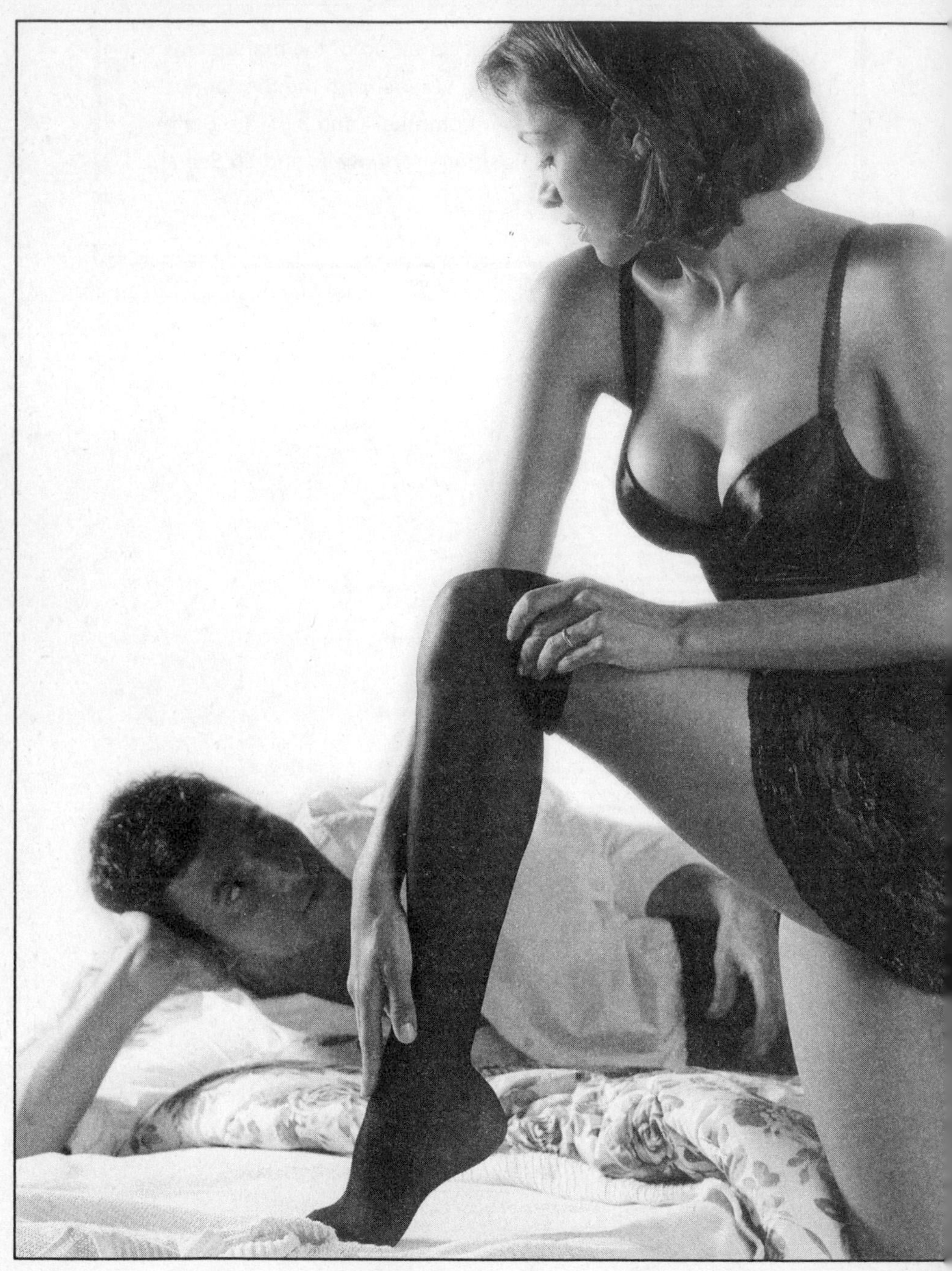

SECRET #9

Indulge Your Fantasies

An improper mind is a perpetual feast.

—LOGAN PEARSALL SMITH
Afterthoughts

Fantasizing about sex is common. Nearly everyone entertains some sort of sexual fantasy life, some outlet for desires that may be impossible, dangerous or otherwise unwise to fulfill. What's so great about fantasy is that there are no restrictions, only possibilities. Allowing yourself to entertain such imaginings can be very freeing. And exploring the deeper meaning of your fantasies can teach you a lot about yourself—what you need more of, what you fear, what parts of you are longing to emerge.

Even if they seem like so much wasted energy to you, fantasies can actually be beneficial. Your fantasies can help you work through restrictions imposed by social norms, and make it possible for you to experience yourself in sexual adventures you might not otherwise experience. Erotic fantasies can also help you dissolve internal barriers, such as insecurities, guilt, fear, or sexual inhibitions. They can even enhance actual sexual encounters by increasing your sexual appetite and intensifying arousal. Research suggests that those with rich fantasy lives enjoy more active and healthy sex lives with their partners.

Some people never have sexual fantasies. Others entertain them frequently. It's probably safe to say that most of us have them more than once a day. Fantasies can come at any time—while we're at work, in church, on the commute home, and, of course, while making love. Some are fully realized stories, others mental snapshots of a scene or desirable individual. Some may be fleeting, but there are some sexual fantasies we replay month after month, year after year.

Although fantasizing is common, few of us ever share our sexual fantasies with our intimate other. We're afraid we'll be judged or ridiculed or worse. No doubt, there are some fantasies that are best kept private. If you know your partner well, you're likely to know which fantasies to keep to yourself and which to share. Yes, we said "share." If the two of you have built up trust, and you feel accepted by your partner, you might want to experiment with letting down your guard and treating each other to the "movies" you create in your erotic imagination. Sharing something so personal builds intimacy and can give you new insight into ways to delight your partner. Just be considerate about keeping to yourself those fantasies or details likely to inflame your partner's jealousy or insecurities. Chances are, you know exactly which ones they are.

Tip: *Having sexual fantasies does not make you immoral or weird. Any fantasy that's occurred to you has probably occurred to other people, at least thematically, even if the details are different. If you replay the fantasy from time to time, without obsessing over it, consider yourself normal.*

Not all fantasies are meant to be shared. Nor do they mean that something is wrong with the marriage. Bonnie and Allen, for instance, had a solid marriage. They had sex regularly, were considerate toward each other, and tender in their lovemaking. Bonnie was happy in her marriage. But that didn't prevent her from replaying an imaginary scene her erotic mind served up to her a few months after their wedding. In her fantasy, she was walking down the street outside their condo, when she noticed a handsome stranger in a leather jacket coming toward her. He gave Bonnie a knowing smile as he passed, then continued along his way. She turned around and followed him, as if drawn by some strange magnet. He continued into a seedier part of town and disappeared into an alley. Bonnie followed. But when she rounded the corner into the alley, he was standing there facing her, his hands on his hips, that same smile on his lips. She melted into his arms. He kissed her, then ripped off her clothes and lifted her up against a brick wall. He entered her and thrust vigorously. The brick felt rough against her bare back. But she was delirious with desire, climaxing again and again. After climaxing himself, the mysterious stranger just walked away without a word.

Bonnie didn't dare tell Allen about her fantasy, for fear of offending him. She tried to repress it, afraid that the fantasy was an indication that she was immoral and unfaithful to her loving husband. But the fantasy would come back again and again, sometimes when she was making love to Allen. Eventually, she realized she could relax and enjoy it without guilt. She was faithful to her husband; the fantasy hadn't changed that.

Bonnie could have decided to share her fantasy with her husband and ask him if he would play it out with her, in one form or another. (It might not be wise, for instance, to have sex in an alley in an unsafe neighborhood, but they could have improvised.) Yet she chose not to share it. There are no rules governing the proper role of fantasy in intimate relationships. It's simply a judgment call.

Another woman might have handled it differently. Sharing a fantasy for the purpose of exploring whether your partner is willing to fulfill it for you can be as fun as it is arousing. Maybe you've been married for a while and you fantasize about going to a pub and picking up a perfect stranger. Maybe he or she is wearing tight leather pants, or something you find even more arousing. Some couples choose to act out these fantasies with each other. Through discussion, they learn what kind of "get-up" would turn their partner on, and they make a date to do the role play. On the appointed evening, they dress in keeping with the fantasy, drive separate cars to an area pub, and act the part of strangers meeting, flirting and deciding to have a fling. Sometimes, the tryst takes place in a roadside motel, just to add to more of a sense of "illicit" sex. Couples who've played in this way say it has created some of the most exciting sex in their lives.

Other common fantasy play scenes include:

—sex with one partner playing an authority figure

—forced sex, with one partner emotionally overpowering the other

—sex for money, with one partner as a prostitute or gigolo

—BDSM play (see Chapter 10)

—one partner wearing a mask, wig or uniform

According to a survey conducted by Yankelovich Partners, approximately one in three American adults report participating in role playing with their partner. The survey found this practice higher among single people in sexual relationships than married people, and higher among those who did not complete high school than those with postgraduate degrees. If you'd like to explore this realm with your partner, you may want to start slowly. Begin by talking about whether the two of you want to share fantasies. Make sure that you're both interested, and that you are both willing to proceed with trust, respect and goodwill. Agree not to laugh or disapprove of what is revealed. Remind each other that entertaining a fantasy does not necessarily indicate a desire to live it out in real life. This will help you create the kind of emotional safety that makes it easier to share your deepest fantasies.

After the groundwork has been set, you may want to start by talking about fantasies that involve your lover. Talk about times you've wanted to have sex with your partner, but didn't find the opening for sexual activity (e.g., Remember when we went to that barbecue last month at Don and Linda's house?). Discuss new settings for sex or activities that you've thought about trying together. Ask "If . . ." questions, like, "If I showed up at your work tomorrow with only a trench coat on, what would you do?"

Considering other people's fantasies can also help break the ice. Get a book of erotic fiction or look over the letters section in an erotic magazine. See if any stories, situations, characters or elements inspire you.

You can also do a little writing of your own. Create an imaginary script for an erotic film together using characters besides yourselves, or inserting yourselves into the action. Or you can keep the process fun by making a game of it. Play "Strip Poker" with layers of the imagination rather than clothing at stake. Try "Truth or Dare" with questions and dares that relate to your fantasies. Take it slowly at first—and don't let one partner get too far ahead of the other in terms of revelation. An imbalance could lead to one partner feeling exposed or manipulated. Try to keep the sharing equal.

And promise yourself that you will never leave a fantasy-sharing session mad or confused. If you notice yourself feeling jealous, disapproving or contemptuous of your partner, stop and talk your feelings through. Reaffirm your affection, respect and commitment to one another. Remind yourselves that the reality of your relationship is more important than anything that goes on in your fantasy worlds.

Fantasy sharing will likely feel a little awkward at first. And a little strange. You may be hearing things from your partner that you never expected. Instead of being judgmental, do your best to cherish and trust the intimacy of the moment. Listen and learn to appreciate the titillation your partner feels from the fantasy.

As you come to understand each other's sexual imaginations, you can even begin to create fantasies for one another. Or do a fantasy relay, with one of you starting the story, then passing the baton to the other to continue it. Sharing sexual activity like heavy petting or mutual masturbation during fantasy can also help escalate the action, increase pleasure and deepen the connections you're forging.

Playing Out Your Fantasies Together

Acting out your fantasies represents another leap of faith for a couple. Something that seems exciting and magical in the imagination can be downright silly or mundane when translated into the physical. Some fantasies may be dangerous to act out. Still, the potential rewards are significant. Many couples report experiencing the hottest sex of their lives while living out a fantasy scene. The intimacy can be just as intense, with partners establishing powerful bonds between previously hidden aspects of their personalities. Fantasy play can also be just plain fun.

Should you give fantasy play a try? There's no pat answer for everyone. But here's a general rule: if it feels good at all levels of your being, go ahead. If it makes you feel compromised, stop.

If you decide to go ahead with it, talk to your partner first about the need for establishing some ground rules. Decide in advance what either of you will do if you want to halt the action because it is becoming uncomfortable.

The lengths you go to reenact a fantasy are up to you and your partner. On the mild side, are those who "dress the part" at an intimate dinner at home. On the wild side, are those who devote an entire room of the home to the props, accessories and apparatus that facilitate the acting out of particular avenues of fantasy. Lovers who are excited by the idea of bondage, for instance, may install wall harnesses, while another couple may decide that the perfect setting for their fantasies is an upscale in-home spa with hot tub and sauna, a place where they can pamper each other and themselves.

Using Fantasy to Improve Your Sex Life

If you find yourself unable to be as free in your sexuality as you'd like, or you would like to feel more confident as a lover, you can use your fantasies, or active imagination, to help. If you "picture" yourself a certain way, and keep feeding your brain the same picture over and over again, your behavior will change to fit the picture. This is the same visualization technique that, say, pro athletes use to improve their game.

First, find a place where you will be undisturbed for twenty minutes. Take the phone off the hook if it is likely to disturb you. Loosen any tight clothing and allow yourself to relax. Try tensing and relaxing each part of your body at least once, so that you can relax deeply. The more you relax, the greater your concentration and the more powerful the results.

Then picture yourself as the kind of lover you want to be. Do you have trouble sexually asserting yourself? Imagine a scene in which you communicate effectively and your partner gives you what you want. Does orgasm still elude you during intercourse? Fantasize about an encounter with your lover, in a setting and lovemaking position that turns you on the most. Lie back and imagine coming to orgasm again and again. Don't skimp on the details or restrict yourself in any way—let your mind take you where you need to go. Allow this hidden part of you the freedom and loving attention it needs to become integrated into your way of being.

If you really want to see the behavior change, do this visualization exercise at least once a day for two weeks.

Question: Are there circumstances under which a fantasy can be harmful?

For the most part, sexual fantasies are normal and healthy. But if you become so obsessed by a particular fantasy that it detracts from your ability to enjoy actual sexual relations, the fantasy may be doing more harm than good. If you find yourself overtaken by an unpleasant or disturbing fantasy, don't repress it. Let it play out. You may want to write it down, to give it full expression. Then seek to discover what's behind it. Ask yourself what it might symbolize. The fantasy may be a way some hidden part of you is trying to get your attention, because there is something you need to become more whole. If these methods don't help you transform the disturbing fantasy into constructive understanding of what you need to grow, seek out the help of a competent therapist.

Common Sexual Fantasies

Our fantasies are as unique as we are. Still, there are common themes. Here's a list of some of the most prevalent:

- Sex in an unusual or exotic setting
- Sex in an everyday setting, like the office
- A sexual encounter based on something seen in the media
- Sexual experimentation
- "Forbidden" types of sex

- Sex in a forbidden place
- Sensuous, romantic sex
- Reliving a past sexual experience
- Engaging in sex for money
- Sex employing special devices or props
- Sex with multiple partners
- Sex with your own partner
- Watching your partner have sex with someone else
- Sex with an ex-partner
- Sex with a new partner, such as:

  —a friend or co-worker

  —a celebrity or world leader

  —someone you see during the morning commute

  —a stranger or masked partner

  —someone in uniform such as a nurse or police officer

  —someone physically or emotionally dominating

  —someone you physically or emotionally dominate

  —someone who finds you irresistible

  —someone from another race or culture

  —someone of the same gender

  —a virgin or someone performing a specific act for the first time

  —someone who gets you to perform a specific act for the first time

If you'd like to see a visual presentation of the material in this chapter, refer to the following videos from the Sinclair Intimacy Institute Video Library: Fantasy—The Better Sex Fantasy Series, Volumes 4-7: *Exploring Sexual Fantasies, Sharing Sexual Fantasies, Acting Out Sexual Fantasies, Advanced Sexual Fantasies,* and *The Erotic Guide to Sexual Fantasies for Lovers.*

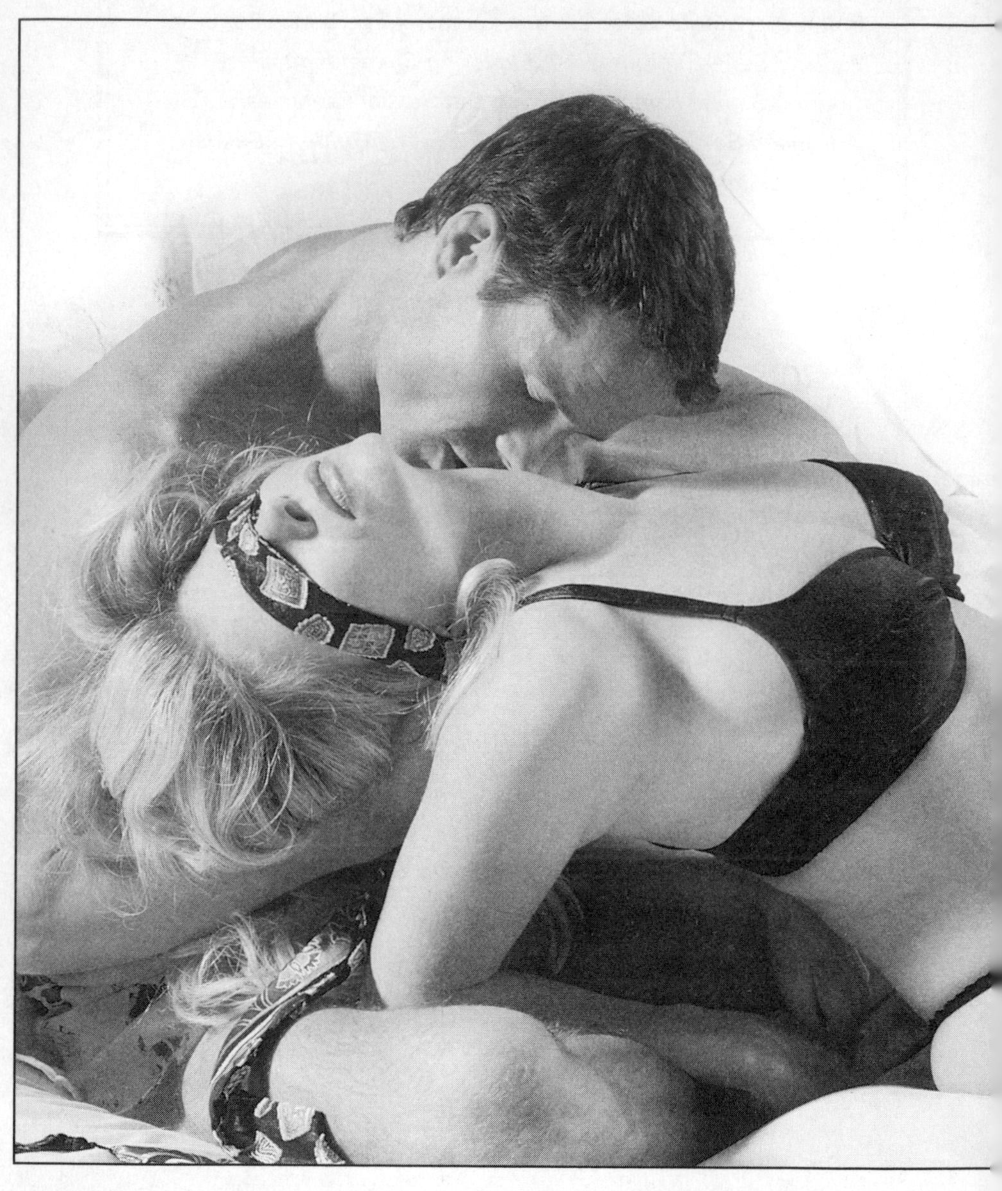

Secret #10

Explore the "Forbidden" Pleasures

Graze on my lips; and if these hills be dry, stray lower, where the pleasant fountains lie.

—Shakespeare
Venus and Adonis

Some people maintain that anything short of intercourse is not "sex." When you consider the actual sexual behavior of American adults, that's far too limited a definition. While intercourse remains the staple of sexual intimacy for most couples, there is a lot more than that going on in American bedrooms. Oral sex and even anal sex are no longer considered deviant behavior. Nor are they the last word on intimate acts couples enjoy in addition to intercourse. We'll touch on those realms later in this chapter.

In "Sex in America," a 1992 University of Chicago survey of sexual behavior, oral sex—which includes fellatio (oral stimulation of the penis) and cunnilingus (oral stimulation of the vulva or clitoris)—

ranked third on a list of sex acts the study's 3,500 respondents preferred. A survey of sexual activity two years later found that one-quarter of all heterosexual adults have engaged, at least once, in anal intercourse. Another survey estimated that about 10 percent of heterosexual couples have anal intercourse once a year.

Of course, it's up to you to decide whether either or both of these sexual acts are right for you. That's a choice you alone can make. Then discuss your feelings with your partner. A loving partner will not persist in trying to persuade you to do something you absolutely do not want to do. By the same token, if your partner feels strongly about experimenting with a particular sexual act, you may be open to trying it just once to see if your experience of the act is different than your ideas about it. That's entirely your call. You have to decide what your "bottom line" is and stick to it, or the resentment is bound to spill out and come between you. It's one thing to "stretch" beyond your comfort zone in an effort to please your partner. That's healthy. It's entirely another thing to treat yourself as if your preferences—or needs—come second. That's unhealthy and won't serve the relationship over the long run. If you don't come first with yourself, you may be sending your partner a signal that it's okay to treat you with the same level of disregard.

With that said, here's the scoop on alternatives to intercourse. The techniques below can help make your forays into the "forbidden zone" as pleasurable as they are exciting.

Tip: *Don't be embarrassed about talking to your partner about oral sex. If you'd like to try something new, ask your partner in a respectful way. If there is any lingering reluctance, discuss all the issues involved. Listen attentively to your partner's concerns. Resist arguing each point. Instead, wait until your partner has spoken his or her piece. Explain what you'd like to try, and ask under what conditions your partner would be willing to go along, even if just once to test it out. Don't regard this discussion as an argument you have to win at all costs, but as a chance to better understand one another. Remain positive and respectful and you are likely to reach a satisfactory resolution for both of you. Keep in mind, too, that reluctance may mask embarrassment, or performance anxiety. If you suspect that's the case here, provide loving encouragement. And don't forget your sense of humor. Be sure to let your partner know that there's no pressure on either of you to bring the other to orgasm orally.*

The Lowdown on "Going Down"

Oral sex has probably been practiced for as long as there have been male and female bodies. The *Kama Sutra*, a book Indian religious scholars compiled and first published over 1,500 years ago, depicts dozens of techniques for oral pleasuring. The ancient erotic text portrays this approach to lovemaking as an important element for partners wishing to establish a loving relationship. Here in the West, oral sex was frowned upon (at least in polite society) until this century. Attitudes about it have changed radically in recent decades. Many women have become as assertive about asking for oral pleasuring as men.

Even though attitudes have relaxed, some individuals remain apprehensive about oral sex. If you count yourself among that crowd, yet remain open to trying it, these techniques may increase your comfort level.

Learning to Love Oral Pleasuring

Oral sex is one of the most intimate sexual activities a couple can engage in. It can provide intense visual stimulation, as well as physical pleasure. Approach it as an act of love, trust, and reverence—and one that provides great pleasure—and you will be richly rewarded.

If you are new to oral sex and a little nervous, you might want to spend some time on your own getting comfortable with the idea of it. Being on the receiving end of oral sex can mean opening yourself up in a manner that can challenge your modesty and sense of self-protection. To help you overcome any apprehensions, find some place where you can have privacy and close the door. Sit down on a chair or lie down and ease open your legs. As you leave them open, close your eyes and imagine your lover's mouth between them. Then sense how that feels in your body. Does it make you tense? Aroused? If you feel tense, gently ask yourself why. What concerns you the most? Listen to yourself and honor your feelings. You may want to discuss them with your partner at an appropriate time.

If the idea arouses you, it's a good idea to keep the fantasy going while you reach your hand down to stimulate yourself manually.

Pretend that it is your lover's tongue and acquaint yourself with the kind of stimulation you like. Do you prefer light and subtle, up and down, vigorous and fast? By probing with your hand, you can map out your pleasure zones. This way you will be much more prepared to tell your partner what you like.

The Art of Oral Pleasuring

Furnishing oral pleasure entails an intricate dance, with no music providing direction or tempo. Each person has his or her own preferences, and your partner will be your best teacher. Still, it's helpful to know a range of techniques so you can offer options and enjoy your own artistry.

As you experiment with oral pleasuring, remember to maintain more than just physical contact throughout the experience. This can be a little tricky with fellatio and cunnilingus. But with some practice, it is possible to focus on what you're doing and stay in contact—which may include eye contact—with your partner. And if you're new to oral sex with each other, by all means, alternate pleasuring your partner with pauses where you stop to ask what feels good, what doesn't, and what he or she wants next.

Cunnilingus: Tips for Men

The clitoris serves as the focal point for cunnilingus. But most women still appreciate having the whole area stimulated. This includes the inside of the thighs, especially the upper thighs. Many women have been taught that "a lady sits with her thighs held tightly together" so it may feel strange at first for a woman to open her legs and keep them open. Gentle, loving strokes that help relax a woman's thighs may prepare her to experience even greater pleasure from oral stimulation.

Men, you may want to start by gently stroking both the top and underside of your partner's thighs. As the thighs open, "reward" them with kisses, loving licks, even little puffs of air. The interior of a woman's thigh is as tender as it is sensitive, so the experience can be exquisite for both of you. It will also make her vulva anticipate your touch.

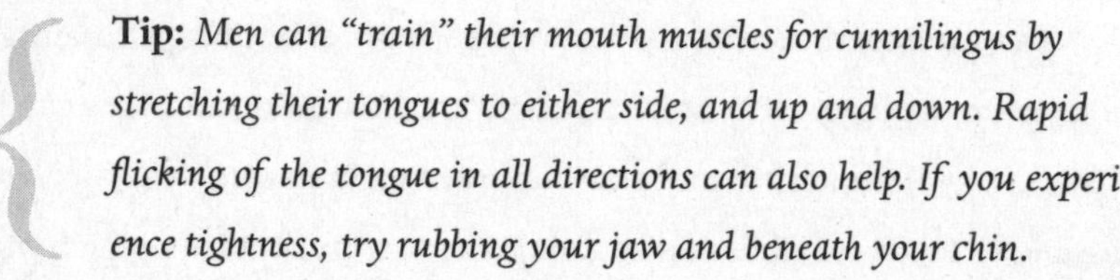

Tip: *Men can "train" their mouth muscles for cunnilingus by stretching their tongues to either side, and up and down. Rapid flicking of the tongue in all directions can also help. If you experience tightness, try rubbing your jaw and beneath your chin.*

Then shift your attention to the outer labia, which will also excite the rest of the vagina. Licking and gently kneading the outer labia between your thumb and index finger for a few minutes will encourage it to send favorable reports to the interior. You may want to ask for your partner's blessing before proceeding further. Many women fear the loss of control in opening themselves up for oral sex. Letting her know that she remains in command of her own safety and pleasure can help her feel safer—and sexier.

When you and your partner are ready to proceed, gently part the outer labia with your fingers. Inside, you'll find the inner labia, clitoris, urethral and vaginal opening. At this point, many men will head straight for the clitoris. But attending to the rest of the vulva can make the experience even more pleasurable for most women. Licking around the lips of the inner labia can feel delicious. Tracing your tongue around the outside of the urethra and on the outside and inside of the vagina may also prove to be quite pleasing. These moves can also build anticipation for clitoral stimulation.

Because the clitoris is intensely sensitive, it should be approached with tender loving care. Although women's preferences vary, it's usually not a good idea to provide direct stimulation at first. Forget about the kind of touch you enjoy when she stimulates your penis. Seek to discover what she likes. Chances are, it will be very different than what you like. Because of the extreme concentration of nerve endings there, the clitoris can actually become overstimulated through excessive direct contact. Realize, also that preferences regarding clitoral stimulation also vary from woman to woman.

Paying attention to the clitoral hood—the small fold of skin that covers the clitoris—may be just the place to start. Gently licking downward, upward, across and/or with a variety of swirls and patterns over the clitoral hood may provide about as much stimulation as she can take. You can also try humming on it, or gently taking it inside your mouth and sucking. Or try using your tongue to "write" her name on it—or yours. Tell her what you're doing and she'll laugh with delight.

You can also try all of these techniques directly on the clitoris by softly pushing back the clitoral hood with your fingers. Be extra gentle here, starting with the kind of touch that's almost "too light to feel." Don't worry, your partner will feel it. As you experiment, do your best to stay attuned to her. Look up from time to time to gaze into her eyes. This can not only help you figure out what's most pleasurable, it may also be a real turn-on for her. Locking eyes with you, as you use your mouth to please her, may increase her love and appreciation for you, and make her more deeply aroused.

It's also a good idea to pause from time to time, and encourage her to tell you or show you exactly what she likes. Be sure to offer her a variety of possibilities, with regard to different levels of pressure and speed. The more moves in your repertoire the better. The clitoris is so sensitive that prolonged stimulation by any one technique or motion can prove irritating. Most women prefer a variety of sensations performed at different speeds and pressures.

Alternating clitoral stimulation with attention to her other erogenous zones can help heighten her pleasure. Try tracing your tongue from the clitoris down to the vagina, then back again, pausing to swirl your tongue around the inside of the vagina before returning. Varying the stimulation like this often feels wonderful for most women. Your tongue may appreciate it, too, because repeating the same motion again and again can be tiring.

Don't be afraid to add manual stimulation. Easing a finger into her vagina and touching the "G-spot" while stimulating her clitoris with your tongue can send your lover over the edge of pleasure to orgasm. Just remember, pleasure—not orgasm—is the only goal of cunnilingus. In fact, putting too much emphasis on climax can detract from the experience for both of you. Given the intimacy, pleasure and goodwill it creates, cunnilingus serves as an end unto itself.

Tip: *Lovers who approach oral sex with enthusiasm score big with their partners. That's easy for some people, who just naturally enjoy it. Those who are a little reluctant may find the act more enjoyable if they sweeten their lover's genitals—the man's penis or the woman's outer labia—with whipped cream, or a flavored lubricant that is meant to be eaten. You can find some of these at the drugstore, or at lingerie shops that specialize in erotic adornment.*

The Best Positions for Cunnilingus

Though many couples are familiar with various positions for intercourse, few understand the importance of positioning for cunnilingus. There are a number of positions that will increase the woman's pleasure, while giving the man easy access. The woman could lie on her back, spread her legs and bring her knees up, keeping her feet on the ground. The man would then lie on his stomach, and move in closer, between her legs, until he's within "tongue-reach" of her genitals. The man's access and the woman's pleasure might both improve if the man places a pillow or two under a woman's hips, in a way that brings the angle of her pelvis upward.

Alternately, the woman could place her legs over her lover's shoulders, allowing her partner to raise her up and simultaneously lick her vulva.

Some women prefer to sit in a chair with wide arms, and have the man kneel in front of her. This frees up her hands to pleasure herself or position her lover's hands. The man may want to put pillows under his knees, which may prevent knee pain and make it easier for him to concentrate on his lover.

If the woman likes being in a position where she has more control over the experience, she can ask her lover to lie down, place pillows under his head and neck, and put her vulva right above his face. This allows the woman to move her vulva over his mouth, and control the speed, direction, location and intensity of stimulation. The only problem with this position is that it doesn't let the woman totally relax, and it may prevent her from totally relaxing into her orgasm. The solution to that may be to have the woman lie on her back, cup her hands beneath her buttocks and move her pelvis over her lover's mouth.

"Rear-entry" cunnilingus offers yet another pleasurable variation. The woman kneels in front of her partner and raises her buttocks, allowing her partner access to her vagina. This may be good for the man, too, since constantly licking and flicking the tongue in one direction can easily tire it. If the woman turns around, the man is able to reverse the motion of his tongue, coming in from above instead of below the vagina. If the woman prefers to lie down after a while, the man can get into position by placing his hands on either side of her hips and bending his head down to her vagina.

Fellatio: Tips for Women

Many men and women adore fellatio. It can seem naughty and nice all at once, and it provides the penis with a wide range of pleasurable sensations. And, like cunnilingus, you can't beat it for visual stimulation—

for both partners. Many men love watching their woman perform fellatio, and many women love watching their man respond.

To do it well, a woman needs to relax, attune herself to her man, and begin softly and slowly, especially if the penis is still soft or only semi-erect. A man may prefer more vigorous stimulation when his penis is fully erect, but it won't feel very good on a soft penis.

And just as it's a good idea for the man to help the woman "warm up" for cunnilingus, it's also a good idea for a woman to consider the best way to help her man prepare for greater pleasure. Many men will immediately rise to the occasion at the prospect of fellatio. But that's just as much a function of his vitality level as it is of his arousal. If your man's penis remains soft even after you begin, don't think he's not enjoying your touch—unless he tells you so. The state of his penis is no reflection on your desirability; so don't assume anything. Ask and trust his answer. Taking your time with your lover is a great way to show him that he's worth your time.

Running your fingertips over the head, shaft and scrotum inspires many men to greater heights. You can also gently hold the penis and lightly shake it from side to side to get the blood flowing into it. Blowing on it, or running your hair over the penis can also get you a standing ovation.

Many women enjoy taking a non-erect penis into their mouths. It's a good way to get your lover erect, and a great way to train your mouth to wrap around the penis. After you take him into your mouth, treat him to a variety of different kinds of wet caresses and licks. Explore him. Tease him. Thrill him. Here are some techniques you can try:

- **Head games.** The head or glans of the penis is incredibly sensitive. Tracing your tongue over and around the glans can prove extremely arousing. Then there's the butterfly—drawing an "8" or butterfly shape from the top front of the shaft, over the glans, to the back top of the shaft.

• **Teasing the shaft.** Running your tongue up and down your lover's shaft works wonders for most men. Try concentrating on the area around the large, protruding vein at the front of the shaft, then explore your way around the shaft to find his other sweet spots.

• **Give him a hand.** Grasping the base of your partner's shaft with your palm while working on the rest of his penis with your mouth may be about the nicest handshake he ever receives. Pumping your hand up and down the shaft while you suck on the glans provides an excellent dynamic duo of sensations.

• **Scrotum play.** Gently, very gently, tickling your lover's scrotum with your tongue or fingers adds yet another delightful sensation to the menu.

• **Flicker.** Flicking your tongue over the coronal ridge (the rim that separates the head from the shaft) and the frenulum (the thin strip of skin on the underside of the head) can come as a sweet surprise.

• **Blowing it.** Puffs of air across the head, shaft and scrotum offer a nice alternative sensation. It's also a good way to catch your breath after having his penis in your mouth.

• **Don't forget the perineum** (the thin strip of skin between the scrotum and the anus). Tickling the perineum with lubricated fingertips can provide a nice secondary treat during oral stimulation. Stimulating it with your fingers or a vibrator can also heighten arousal.

• **Deep throating.** Although this is falsely thought to be the "ideal" fellatio technique, few women are able to do this. Just like it sounds, deep throating involves taking your lover's entire penis in and out of your mouth, which for most means getting a good deal of it into your throat without gagging. Obviously, this requires lots of practice and a great deal of relaxation and experimentation with angles. Don't be discouraged if you never quite get it. You can give great fellatio without having to do this.

• **Change is good**. Altering your rhythm and level of pressure as well as your techniques usually makes for more satisfying fellatio. Note your lover's favorite (ask, or just listen for moans and gasps) for the stretch run, going to it and sticking with it until he climaxes.

• **To swallow or not to swallow.** Once your man does climax, the issue arises about what to do with the semen. Some women enjoy swallowing it, and many men encourage this. But if you don't like the taste or feel of semen, don't be shy about spitting it into a towel or removing your mouth from your lover's penis just before he ejaculates. Do what's comfortable for you. Just don't worry about the calories. The average ejaculate contains about four calories, if that.

The Best Positions for Fellatio

There are a few positions that really work for fellatio. Having the man lie on a bed or floor while his lover leans over him is very popular. Couples can also lie in a "69" position while the woman takes the man's penis into her mouth. Still other couples are turned on by the raciness of having the man standing or leaning back against the wall, while his partner kneels before him. Just make sure the woman's knees are resting on a pillow or something comfortable. Whatever position you choose, make sure it's comfortable for both of you. That will help you extend this form of play as long as you would like. And speaking of comfort, men who instinctively place a hand or two on the back of their lover's head during fellatio should be careful not to get too enthusiastic because she could gag or find it difficult to breathe if she doesn't pace herself.

ORAL SEX MYTHS

There's a lot of misinformation about oral sex. Here are some of the most common misconceptions:

There's one "right way" to do it. There's no single effective way to perform cunnilingus or fellatio. Look to your partner's preferences to guide you.

The "69" position is the ultimate. Simultaneous oral stimulation between two partners—or "69ing," as some refer to it—can be a lot of fun. But it can also be a logistical nightmare, with neither partner getting the full attention of the other. That means both end up feeling shortchanged. The "69" is an advanced position, and doesn't always work even for couples who've mastered the other aspects of oral sex.

The only reason to do it is to bring your partner to orgasm. Orgasms are always nice, but there's no rule that says you have to stimulate your partner to orgasm, no matter what sexual act you're engaged in. The same goes for oral sex. Some people just can't achieve climax during oral stimulation, no matter how skilled or determined their partner. And if the process goes on too long, both partners will feel too exhausted or frustrated to do anything else. Oral sex does a great job of tantalizing, providing pleasure and deepening the bond between lovers. Anything beyond that is gravy.

You have to go "deep" to do an adequate job. This is not true whether you're performing oral sex on the man or woman. It's good for women to realize that effective fellatio does not require "deep throating"—the insertion of the entire penis into the mouth and throat. The truth is that pressure, location and timing are much more important to oral stimulation than the depth of insertion.

Cunnilingus is only clitoral. Clitoral stimulation is the main attraction of cunnilingus. But focusing solely on the clitoris can actually cause a woman discomfort. Try getting the whole vagina involved.

You're supposed to do it vigorously from the start. Most men and women enjoy—or even require—a period of gentle stimulation to warm up for oral sex. Help get your partner in the mood by softly licking, stroking and tickling his or her erogenous zones.

"If you love me, you'll swallow." Some women find swallowing their lover's semen unpleasant. Men, realize it's a personal preference that has nothing to do with the woman's degree of love for you. Women, realize that you have the right to ask your partner to let you know when he's about to ejaculate so you can bring him over the edge by stimulating him with your hand.

Oral means "oral only." And "task" and "unpleasant" have no place in the oral sex vocabulary. Actually, oral sex allows for help from the hands, vibrators, or anything else that helps stimulate your lover. Don't get limited by semantics.

Oral sex is easy. Lunchroom braggarts and Hollywood's bedroom scenes would have us believe that oral pleasuring comes quickly and easily. Truth is, like most skills, it requires a lot of practice. The nice thing is that in a loving relationship, practicing oral sex is a lot more fun than hitting backhands or rehearsing an office presentation.

Anal Sex: Making the "End" the Means

The prospect of anal sex provokes strong reactions. Some people regard it as unclean and immoral. Others find defying its taboos exciting, and love the sensations it arouses. If you're interested in initiating anal play, ask your partner whether he or she is interested. You may find you have very different ideas about it, so talk before you act. Don't touch or otherwise stimulate your partner's anus without permission because even a gentle touch can seem like a serious violation of trust.

Acquainting Yourself with Anal Anatomy

Because the anus serves as the body's main waste-disposal corridor, the idea of using it as an organ of penetration may seem outrageous at first. What you might want to consider, however, is that urine flows out of the penis and through the opening in the vulva—yet people don't think twice about inserting one into the other. The other thing the anus has in common with the penis and vagina is that there is a high concentration of nerve endings there, which qualifies it as an erogenous zone. Most of those nerve endings exist around the outside rim of the anus. (This area is a great starting—and for some—ending-point for anal play.)

The inside of the anal rim is surrounded by two powerful, dough-nut shaped sphincter muscles. The inner one is designed to contract and keep anything from entering the body. With practice and patience, it can be coaxed into relaxing. The anus extends only about an inch inside, giving way to the rectum, a tube-like structure that extends for about 5 to 9 inches to the colon, where waste is stored. The interior walls of the rectum are also loaded with nerve endings, making them very sensitive to sensation. The walls are also quite delicate, and can be easily damaged.

In men, the prostate gland sits just below the rectum along the front wall of the anus. About the size of a walnut (at least until it starts growing when men get into their 40s), the prostate is extremely sensitive and can be coaxed into orgasmic contraction.

Tips on Anal Safety

The first and foremost consideration with anal play is safety. Anal sex can cause damage and lead to other health problems if partners are careless. Here are ways to approach anal play responsibly.

- Bathe the anus before engaging in play. It is filled with germs and tiny bits of fecal matter. If any of that gets into the partner's mouth, nostrils or a woman's vagina, it can cause disease. An enema prior to anal play can clean out any fecal matter.

- It is also important to wash your hands, or any sex toy, before and after it comes into contact with the anus. Consider covering the sex toys with condoms, since you can throw them away afterwards and put a fresh one on when you use the toy again.

- File your nails and use something to smooth over any calluses. (Latex gloves will do the trick.) A jagged fingernail or a callused finger can damage the anus and cause your partner great discomfort for weeks to come. Be sure fingers are smooth and clean (and well lubricated) before play begins.

• Wear a condom. Studies indicate that anal sex may transmit sexually transmitted diseases—especially AIDS— more efficiently than any other sexual activity. (If you are in a new relationship and you haven't talked to your partner yet about whether they have any sexual diseases, or have been tested for AIDs, have that discussion now.) For anal intercourse, choose a latex condom covered in a thick water-based lubricant that will leave the condom intact. Oil-based lubricants can cause the condom to deteriorate.

• Lubricate inside the anus, too. The anus requires thick and plentiful lubrication before and during play. Don't rely on the condom's lubrication alone.

• Be gentle. The walls of the anal canal can be easily cut or torn through aggressive thrusting or rushed entry. If the walls have not relaxed enough, you may want to purchase an "anal starter kit," which has three plugs that progressively open the anus.

• Keep the lines of communication wide open. The person on the receiving end of anal stimulation needs to stay in control throughout, and stop the action if something hurts.

• Talk afterwards. Discuss what felt good, whether you'd like to have anal sex again. (If something felt uncomfortable, talk about that, too and what you can change next time. It isn't supposed to hurt, and it won't hurt if done right.) Don't forget to reaffirm your affection for each other afterwards. This is particularly important after engaging in any new sexual activity.

Preparing the Anus for Sex Play

Healthy and pleasurable anal play requires good preparation. The first step, of course, is to make sure you and your partner have talked about anal play and both of you feel good about trying it. (In many couples, one may be more excited about the prospect than the other, but the partner needs to feel okay about it, too.) The next is to create a little ritual around getting ready.

You may want to start with an enema, to clean any fecal matter from the rectum and anus. You may want to follow that with a warm bath. While you are in the tub, try clenching the sphincter muscles, holding the contraction for a few seconds, then easing up. Repeat this exercise until you feel in tune with the muscles and can tell when they are relaxed and contracted. This may help them relax.

When you get out of the bath, make sure your bottom is thoroughly dry. Water is not a good lubricant and can wash away the lubricant you need. It's a good idea at this point for the partner who is penetrating the other's anus (with a finger, sex toy, or penis) to massage the "receiving" partner. This can dissolve tension, make it easier to relax the anal sphincter, and increase the receiver's sense of honor and control, while making him or her more receptive to the pleasurable stimulation to follow.

Just before engaging in anal play, lubricate the anus thoroughly.

Keep the bottle nearby so you can add more as needed. Because this can be messy, you may want to place a bath towel underneath you.

Making Anal Play Pleasurable

The outside of the anus provides a nice starting point for anal play. The perineum—the thin strip of skin stretching from the bottom of the genitals to the top of the anus—will enjoy a gentle, well-lubricated touch. The anal rim may take great pleasure in being softly orbited by a lubricated finger or tongue. A vibrator may also provide pleasure here.

External anal play can be delightful and arousing. That may be as far as some individuals want to go. They may enjoy external touch for its own sake and as a way to enhance the sensations leading to orgasm.

Tip: *There is speculation, but not proof, that the prostate is the male version of the "G-spot." It's rich with nerve endings and can be just as responsive to pleasuring as its female counterpart. Pleasuring the prostate can also bring a man to orgasm. This is not well known, possibly because the male prostate can only be stimulated directly through the anus.*

Men, to stimulate your prostate, use a lubricated finger (you could also protect your finger by wearing a latex glove), and probe for a lump just a few inches on the forward wall of the anus. Try tapping it or stroking it with a "come here" motion, just like you would with the "G-spot"—only reverse the motion. Or use a toy that's specially curved for prostate play. Men who don't realize that they have a "P-spot" come to love it, once they get over their initial nervousness about its placement.

If you and your partner want to proceed to anal penetration, be sure to go very slowly and gently. Again, the anus and rectum are delicate and can be easily damaged.

Vibrators can be great for external and internal anal sex play because they provide nice and constant stimulation, which can help the area relax. Thin dildos or anal plugs or beads can also be enjoyable. Look for toys that are designed for anal play—dildos and plugs should have a flanged or wide base to prevent the plug from slipping or going in too deep. Longer toys usually feature bowed, flexible stems that won't damage the curved walls of the rectum. Remember to cover the toys with a condom, or clean them with hydrogen peroxide before and after anal play.

Interior anal stimulation needs to begin slowly, softly, and shallowly. If done properly, this stage can be very pleasurable and clear the way for deeper penetration. If done improperly, it can cause pain, hurt feelings and make your partner reluctant to ever try it again. Try gently working the tip of a finger inside the anus. The sphincter muscles are likely to clench in response, to keep the finger out. Remain patient and gentle. Slowly, work the finger inside.

Once your partner has gotten comfortable with a finger or two, or a toy, you may want to try a penis. Apply a condom and plenty of lubricant first. Be extra gentle and cautious as you enter, and redouble your communication efforts. The person on the receiving end needs to control the pace, force and depth of penetration at all times, so let him or her call the shots. In fact, the receiver should be the only one moving at first, using the motions of his or her backside to dictate pace, depth and force of the penetration.

Question: My husband enjoyed the first time I played with his anus, but he's worried it means he might be homosexual. What can I do to ease his fears?

Though some fear it will label them as "homosexual," many heterosexual men engage in regular anal stimulation. Some report achieving swift erections and enjoying their most powerful orgasms during anal play. Assure your husband that enjoying anal play does not make him gay or straight, just secure in his pleasures.

Spanking and Other Sexual "Games"

In an ideal world, people's lives and relationships would be harmoniously balanced. Children would learn early how to resolve negative emotions in a constructive way, and grow through the more painful experiences of life into better, more resilient people. And adults wouldn't need to inflict pain on others, or have it inflicted to feel sexual excitement. But this isn't an ideal world. And because the sexual energy is an expression of the life force, unresolved issues in a person's life tend to show up in the bedroom.

Sometimes sexuality is the only outlet for inner conflicts or past trauma. It may also be the avenue through which a person's inner self can express the need for balance. Maybe that's why professional dominatrixes say that their best clients are high-powered business executives. Men who call the shots twelve hours a day, five days a week, are probably just looking to relax and give up control to someone else for a while. When you look at it that way, it makes more sense.

So while sexual practices like bondage & discipline, dominance & submission and sadism & masochism—BDSM—may seem bizarre on the surface, it is not difficult to understand why these practices persist. Who hasn't, at times, felt guilty (and, perhaps, an unconscious desire to be punished), or humiliated, or powerless? Because few people explore these emotions within themselves, there's a certain excitement about re-experiencing this charged internal content in sex play. For some couples, BDSM practices afford a convenient and sexually exciting outlet for these feelings. And some just enjoy the excitement of engaging in sexual play that's at the outer limits of acceptability.

You and your partner may already use elements of BDSM without even realizing it. Talking dirty, teasing, a gentle bite on the neck, or a quick slap on the rear involve emotional elements common in BDSM. When you think about it, almost all positions for intercourse and oral sex involve dominant and submissive postures, with one partner setting the tone and pace, while the other remains relatively passive.

In the last ten years, BDSM play has entered the sexual mainstream. Surveys tell us that millions of people engage in these practices each year. If this realm of sexuality intrigues you, it is possible to explore it without becoming a sexual deviant. Just keep it light and pay attention to those inner messages that warn you when you're about to overstep your own boundaries and violate your integrity, or cause harm to another.

Fantasies serve as an ideal starting place for introducing BDSM into your love life. (See Chapter 9.) If you've both been aroused by describing BDSM dynamics during fantasy play, you may want to try them out in your love life. If the theme has yet to come up, and you're intrigued, by all means, bring it up. You may want to start with something simple, like asking your partner if he or she can bind your hands or feet to the bedpost with silk while he or she provides oral pleasuring. Then talk about whether you want to take this any further.

If you do, just take is slowly. If one partner gets ahead of the other, or if one finds in midstream that he or she is just not turned on, these games can end up sacrificing—instead of increasing—intimacy. So stay in tune with your partner's feelings before, during and after role-play.

If things are going well, you can add some elements of BDSM during intercourse. Choose a position where one partner is on top. The person on top can gently pin down his or her partner's wrists during thrusting. Uttering a few bossy or dominant words can up the ante a little. Now try switching sides, with each of you assuming the opposite role. While one partner will likely tend toward the dominant role ("the top") and the other the submissive ("the bottom"), it's important that each of you know how the other half feels. Many regular BDSM players report regularly switching roles.

It's also vital to understand that the person in the submissive role actually controls the action. Most "tops" usually ask their "bottoms" for permission to proceed before initiating a new activity (e.g., "I'm going to spank you now. You'd like that, wouldn't you?") This helps the submissive partner remain in control of the situation while also building anticipation.

Should things go too far, the "submissive" partner should say so immediately, causing the initiating partner to downshift or back off completely. To this end, couples adopt a special "stop sign"—a phrase or gesture from the submissive partner that signals discomfort. The sign should be easy to say or make and impossible to misinterpret. Choose something other than the word "No" or "Stop" as your special phrase to signal that the action should stop. Also, keep in mind that physical restraints introduced into the play should not keep the "submissive" partner from signaling for a stop. A spoken stop sign is no good if the individual has a scarf across the mouth.

BDSM can be as simple or elaborate as you like. Basic activities include spanking, blindfolding and applying restraints to the hands and/or feet. With spanking, aim for the meaty part of the buttocks, vary the timing and force of the strikes, never hitting so hard that you cause bruising or lasting pain. If you blindfold your partner, make sure he or she is someplace where there's no chance of falling or bumping into something. With restraints, be very careful not to fix them too tightly on wrists or ankles so blood flow isn't cut off and that the cuffs don't dig into the skin. Unless you're a master at tying knots, rope can be tricky to untie quickly if you notice circulation problems. If you use rope, keep a good pair of scissors by the bed. Most sex toy companies now offer restraints made of soft material with Velcro fasteners for easy release.

Also make sure that you never walk away from your lover after you put restraints or a blindfold on him or her. This is not only dangerous, but can seriously undermine trust in a relationship.

If these activities prove fun, you might want to move on to more elaborate scenarios that involve costumes and other toys. Alternately, you can incorporate elements of BDSM into your regular sex play.

If you'd like to see a visual presentation of the material in this chapter, refer to the following videos from the Sinclair Intimacy Institute Video Library: Better Sex Video Series®, Volume 2: *Advanced Sexual Techniques, The guide to Oral Sex, Better Oral Sex Techniques,* and *Forbidden Pleasures.*

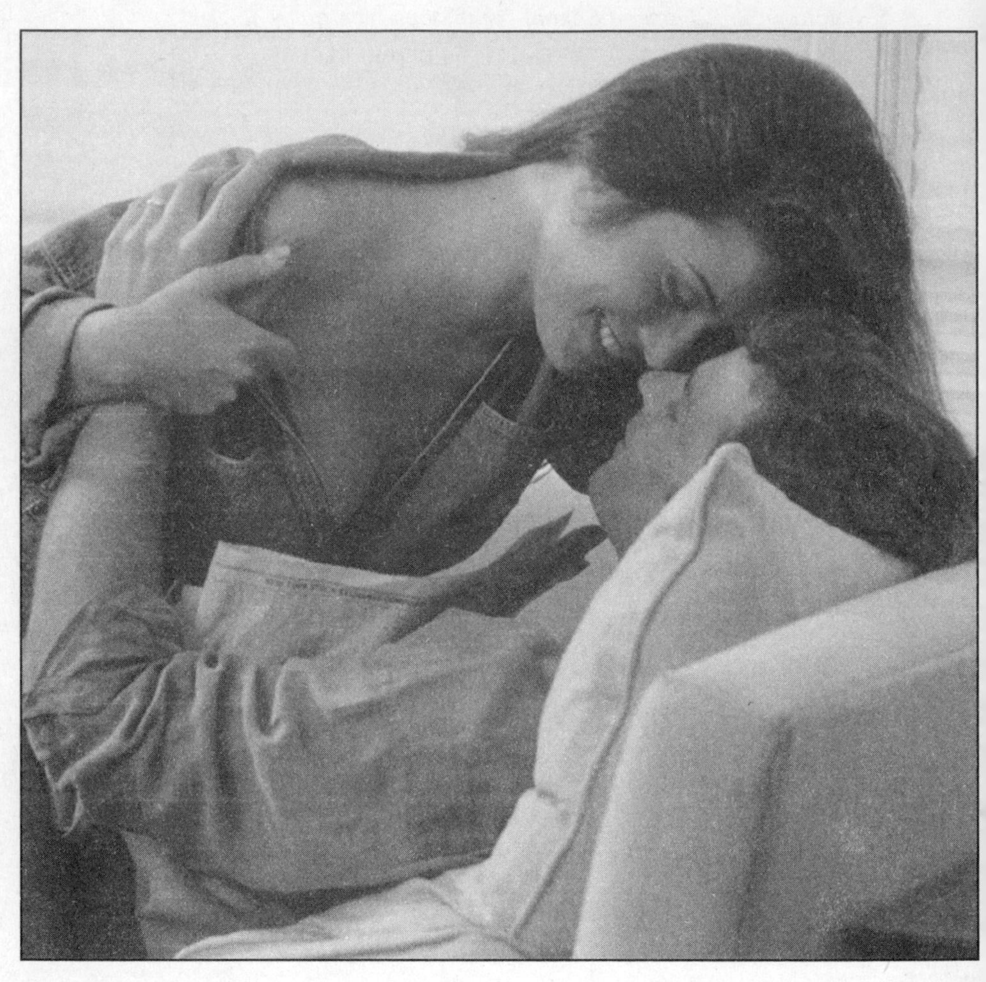

Epilogue

The Art of Making Love

> *One can learn technique, but never feeling, and feeling is the main factor, for the art of giving pleasure is the art of love and devotion.*
>
> —A. Costler, M.D.
> *Encyclopedia of Sexual Knowledge*

You can acquire all the "technical" sexual skills you want, and still not be a great lover. As we have said throughout the book, extraordinary sex is not just physical. That kind of sex is one-dimensional. Truly extraordinary sex engages the intellect, the emotions and the spirit.

How?

You engage the intellect by allowing for plenty of variety in your lovemaking. Spontaneity, rather than routine, becomes the order of the day. As you come to know each other better, you find creative ways to artfully arouse the senses that show your partner you do indeed know what turns him or her on. If your lover is a wine connoisseur, for instance, you might set up "wine-tasting" zones on your body, and set out a basket of bread and water nearby, for cleansing the palate. If your lover is into the martial arts, you might dress for love in a silk kimono, or do naked t'ai chi together to get your energy flowing. By the same token, you'd approach a new mother gently, sensitive to the fact that intercourse might still be painful. You'd take extra time to help a harried executive relax, perhaps giving him or her a foot massage or back rub. Thoughtfulness counts for a lot.

You engage the emotions by approaching your partner with genuine affection, reverence, appreciation and concern for their well-being. These qualities can never be faked or forced. Heartfulness—as well as its absence—is always apparent.

You engage the spirit by your willingness to reveal yourself, to get as naked emotionally as you do physically, and to let go of self-defenses that serve as barriers to intimacy. When you can really attune yourself to your lover, and he or she to you, hearts, minds and bodies merge into an expansive union, one that fills hungers beyond the physical.

This is the way of love. Love is not afraid to explore new avenues of pleasure, even as it appreciates what is. It is not afraid to risk, even as it is careful to conserve what it has. It knows that it is boundless and full, that there are countless ways to express it and infinite varieties of pleasure to be had by those who honor its ways.

APPENDIX A

Eating for Potency and Pleasure

The back pages of many magazines are filled with advertisements for sexual aids and "aphrodisiacs"—usually herbal supplements that claim to restore youthful sexual vigor. However, the best way to increase sexual health and energy is to stick to a balanced diet that's high in vegetables, fruits, whole grains and lean meats, and low in sugars, fats and processed foods. That's the surest bet for enhancing day-to-day sexual functioning and maintaining your youth over the years.

If you're observant, you have probably noticed that you don't feel much like having sex, or doing anything energetic, right after you've eaten rich, fatty foods or overindulged in junk foods. It can take more energy to digest unhealthy foods than whole grains and vegetables, and what's worse, poorer-grade foods don't replace the energy they've taken during digestion. Eating "cleaner" will give each of you more stamina. In men, the relationship between a diet and sexual functioning is even more pronounced. The same eating habits that lead to high cholesterol—which can bring on heart disease and high blood pressure—can also lead to erection problems, since the narrowing of the arteries associated with heart disease also affects blood flow to the penis.

Exercise is just as important as a healthy diet if you want to maintain your good looks and vitality. With good habits like these, you won't need to waste your money on "miracle" products.

APPENDIX B

Tips for Lovers in Special Circumstances

Lovers come in all sizes, ages and with different physical circumstances. Sometimes, these present special challenges to the intimate relationship, or the lovemaking itself. With a little creativity, these challenges can be surmounted. Love is always stronger than the obstacles.

Pregnant Couples

Couples often worry that sex during pregnancy might harm the baby. In a normal pregnancy, lovemaking is usually considered safe. In fact, sex can go a long way toward easing the fears and tension stirred up by this transition into family life. That's not to say that concerns about sex during pregnancy aren't legitimate. Talk to your doctor about precautions you might want to take during different stages of pregnancy.

Even though most women are able to make love during the course of pregnancy, that doesn't mean they'll always want to. Because of all the hormonal changes during pregnancy, women go through many ebbs and flows of desire during the course of pregnancy. During the first trimester, women may experience morning sickness, exhaustion and a reduction in sex drive. Fortunately for their partners, in the second trimester women often experience an increase in sex drive.

For some, sexual desire even climbs to an all-time high. And then in the third trimester— the final three months of pregnancy—desire often wanes again as physical discomfort and belly size increase.

According to the Kinsey Institute's "New Report on Sex," by June M. Reinisch, PhD. and Ruth Beasley, M.L.S., many couples refrain from sex toward the end of the third trimester because the contractions of orgasm can start the contractions of childbirth. (Some midwives actually recommend intercourse as a natural way to induce labor when the baby has come to term.)

Other couples continue to have sex through the pregnancy. If you'd like to, get your doctor's OK first. Listen to your own intuition as well about what feels right for you and the baby. If going ahead with intercourse feels okay to you, do avoid all sexual positions that place pressure on the woman's stomach. Try a spooning or rear-entry position. Also avoid deep thrusting.

After childbirth, it may take several months for a woman's vaginal tissues to heal. She may experience pain if she tries to rush back into sex, especially if she has had an episiotomy (a small surgical incision to widen the vaginal opening) or suffered a vaginal tear during birth. She may also experience a decrease in lubrication caused by the hormonal changes associated with breast-feeding. A wane in desire is also very likely, because of the physical demands of caring for a newborn.

No matter what stage of pregnancy or postpregnancy they find themselves in, couples can stay sexually connected through erotic touching, massage, and mutual masturbation, if they wish to refrain from intercourse.

Couples with Young Children

It is especially challenging for parents of young children to find the time, energy and privacy for intimate time. These guidelines can help:

• **Keep sex a priority.** Though it often falls to the bottom of the list, intimate time with each other is essential to the health and happiness of the whole family. Make private time a priority on your schedule.

• **Set boundaries.** Put a lock on your bedroom door so that the kids don't wander in when you're making love. Let them know that your bedroom is your special space, just like their bedrooms are for them.

• **Don't deny your sexual rhythms.** Many couples get stuck in a rut—only making love late at night when the kids are asleep (and when they are usually exhausted). Hire a babysitter to take them to Saturday matinees or make regular playdates for them with their grandparents. Or work out trades with a playmate's family. Chances are the kids will be as thrilled with their special daytime activities as you are with yours.

Divorced People in a New Relationship

People who find romance after a divorce have an opportunity to make a fresh start and define love on their own terms. They're older, wiser and better equipped to find what they want—in life and in bed. These suggestions can help you ease into intimacy with a new partner:

• **Give yourself sufficient time to let go of old hurts and anger, and to heal your heart, before you jump into a new relationship.**

Otherwise, you risk repeating the dynamics that caused your prior relationship to sour. Then do your best to make a new start, without bringing unfinished business with your old spouse into the new relationship.

• **Don't expect your new partner to have the same needs, preferences or boundaries as your ex did.** Everyone is different sexually. Stay open and pay attention, so that you can discover what pleases and excites this new partner.

• **Open yourself to the "new."** Remember things you enjoyed when you were younger that your ex insisted on deleting from your sexual repertoire. Play with new games and toys. Experiment. You've got a new chance at happiness, so have some fun with it.

Active Seniors

Clear your mind of any false condition that sex is only for the young. Many couples continue to have wonderful sexual experiences well into their golden years. Older couples have some advantages over youthful ones. Individuals are more likely to understand their own needs and desires they know each other well, and they have a lifetime of sexual experience to draw on.

That said, it's unrealistic to expect sex at 75 to be just like it was at 25. Around the age of 40, men and women start to undergo physical changes that affect their sexuality. Older woman may experience a decrease in vaginal lubrication, so find a lubricant that works for you. Orgasms may be less intense.

Men may find that their erections are not as firm and reliable as they were in their younger days. Like women, they may also notice that their orgasms are less intense. As men age, they may need a longer rest period between ejaculations. In these cases, an erection ring can help.

Although gradual changes are normal, if you experience dramatic changes in your sexual response as you get older, see your doctor. You want to make sure that the dramatic change isn't an indication of a serious medical problem.

Couples who gracefully navigate these changes in their sexuality as they age tend to have excellent communication, as well as the willingness to adapt certain practices—or adopt new ones—to meet their needs. They may find it helpful, for instance, to use more lubrication than before, engage in more oral and manual stimulation, and explore new forms of sexual stimulation such as sex toys, fantasy play or erotic videos. (The Sinclair videos that address sexuality for mature lovers include *Couples Guide to Great Sex Over 40*, Vol. 1 & 2, *Better Sex for a Lifetime*, Vol. 1 & 2, *Sex After 50, A Man's Guide to Stronger Erections*, and *Menopause and Beyond.*)

When active seniors approach the changes in their sexuality with the right spirit, there's no reason that their intimate time together can't become even more golden as the years go on.

Those Overcoming Sexual Trauma

Individuals who have experienced sexual trauma—whether through molestation, sexual abuse or rape—can ultimately overcome its destructive impact, with the right kind of help. That can take time. While there is nothing more healing than the love of a patient, caring and accepting partner, a therapist's help is almost always necessary. That's because many abuse victims develop strong subconscious defenses, and negative attitudes about sexuality and themselves. These subconscious beliefs can interfere with their ability to experience pleasure in the sexual act, make them feel unworthy of the love of their partner, or cause them to "split" love and sex—meaning they find it difficult for them to have sexual feelings toward someone they love.

Until the individual is able to fully heal from the trauma, he or she may experience inhibited desire, guilt, anxiety, or waves of intense anger. Spacing out—disassociating the mind from the body—during sex is also common.

Because the pain of this kind of trauma is so intense, it can lead to self-destructive coping strategies, such as alcohol abuse, drug abuse or sexual addiction. That's why the assistance of a credentialed counselor who is specifically trained to work with victims of sexual abuse is often necessary. A therapist can help couples get to the root of the difficulties in their intimate relationship, advise them on coping strategies, and guide them through the healing process. It's often helpful for the partner who has not experienced sexual abuse to go for counseling, too, or join a support group for spouses in the same situation.

The individual who has experienced the abuse may find that talk therapy is a safe way to start the healing process. But it may not go far enough. Body-based psychotherapies, such as Bioenergetics, Core Energetics and the Rubenfeld Synergy Method, can help the victim contact and release trauma still held in the body. Other hands-on healing modalities, such as therapeutic massage, or spiritual healing, can also speed the healing process and make it easier for the victim to reconnect with pleasurable feelings in the body.

Other modalities that may be helpful include:

- Expressive therapies, such as dance, music or art therapy

- Oriental arts such as t'ai chi or qi gong

- Bodywork such as The Feldenkrais Method, a movement retraining system that helps people improve posture and move with a new lightness; or Jin Shin Jitsu, which works with pressure points to help release repressed emotions and restore well-being

- Guided imagery, which can be used to help people identify and overcome subconscious obstacles and inhibitions

- Yoga, which decreases stress, and brings harmony to body and mind

Couples with Chronic Marital Problems

While mutually fulfilling sex can deepen bonds in a healthy relationship, don't expect it to compensate for serious marital rifts. If your own efforts to resolve difficulties don't bring much change, you may want to consider engaging a qualified marriage and family counselor, or, in certain specific situations, a qualified sex therapist. Just be very selective because a therapist not suited to your needs can make matters worse. That's why it's a good idea to check references, and to have an introductory visit with several possible counselors before choosing one you both like. One good referral source for qualified counselors is the American Association of Sex Educators, Counselors and Therapists. To learn more about the organization, Call 804-644-3288, or visit the website at www.aacest.org.

Here are some red flags that a relationship is in danger:

- There are chronic disagreements about sex.

- Criticism dominates communication.

- Negative emotions are so strong, couples refuse to touch each other in a nurturing way.

- Attempts to improve the sexual relationship lead to arguments and increase distance between partners.

- One or both partners engage in addictive behaviors such as drinking too much, drug abuse, overeating, workaholism, or compulsive shopping, etc.

- The residual affects of sexual trauma make it difficult or impossible for that individual to sustain a healthy sex life.

- Chronic sexual dysfunction.

- Inability to regain trust after an affair.

BIBLIOGRAPHY

Barbach, Lonnie. *Fifty Ways to Please Your Lover: While You Please Yourself.* New York: Dutton, 1997.

Barbach, Lonnie. *For Yourself: The Fulfillment of Female Sexuality* (Newly Revised and Updated). New York: Penguin Putnam, Inc., 2000.

Bass, Ellen, and Lauren Davis. *The Courage to Heal: A Guide for Women Survivors of Sexual Abuse.* New York: Harper Perennial, 1994.

Bechtel, Stefan, Laurence Roy Stains, and the editors of Men's Health books. *Sex: A Man's Guide.* Emmaus: Rodale Press, Inc., 1996.

Blank, Joani, and Ann Whidden. *Good Vibrations: The New Complete Guide to Vibrators.* Revised edition. San Francisco: Down There Press, 2000.

Chalker, Rebecca. *The Clitoral Truth: The Secret World at Your Fingertips.* New York: Seven Stories Press, 2000.

Chia, Mantak, and Douglas Abrams. *The Multi-Orgasmic Man: Sexual Secrets Every Man Should Know.* San Francisco: HarperSanFrancisco, 1996.

Comfort, Alex, M.D. *The New Joy of Sex: A Gourmet Guide to Lovemaking in the Nineties.* New York: Pocket Books, 1991.

Greene, Robert. *The Art of Seduction.* Produced by Joost Elffers. New York: Viking, 2001.

Heiman, Julia R., and Joseph LoPiccolo. *Becoming Orgasmic: A Sexual and Personal Growth Program for Women.* New York: Fireside / Simon & Schuster, 1988.

Hite, Shere. *Women Are Revolutionary Agents of Change: The Hite Reports and Beyond.* Madison: University of Wisconsin Press, 1994.

Hooper, Anne. *Anne Hooper's Pocket Kama Sutra: A New Guide to the Ancient Arts of Love.* New York: DK Publishing, Inc., 1996.

Inkeles, Gordon, and Murray Todris. *The Art of Sensual Massage.* New York: Simon & Schuster, 1972.

Ladas, Alice Kahn, Beverly Whipple, and John D. Perry. *The G Spot and Other Discoveries about Human Sexuality.* New York: Dell Publishing, 1982.

Lloyd-Elliott, Martin. *Secrets of Sexual Body Language.* Berkeley: Ulysses Press, 1994.

Newman, Felice. *The Whole Lesbian Sex Book: A Passionate Guide for All of Us.* SanFrancisco: Cleis Press, 1999.

Reinisch, June M., and Ruth Beasley. *The Kinsey Institute New Report on Sex.* New York: St. Martin's Press, 1991.

Rosenthal, Saul H., M.D. *The New Sex Over 40.* New York: J P Tarcher, 1999.

Scantling, Sandra R., Psy.D., Browder, Sue Ellin. *Ordinary Women, Extraordinary Sex.* New York: Dutton/Plume, 1994.

Scantling, Sandra R., Psy.D. *Extraordinary Sex Now.* New York: Doubleday, 1998.

Slowinksi, Julian, Milsten, Richard. *The Sexual Male: Problems and Solutions.* New York: W.W. Norton & Company, Inc., 1999.

Stubbs, Kenneth Ray, Saulnier, Louise-Andree, Spencer, Kyle. *Erotic Massage: The Touch of Love.* Tucson: Secret Garden Publishing, 1991.

Swift, Rachel. *How to Have an Orgasm as Often as You Want.* New York: Carroll & Graf Publishers, Inc., 1993.

Tisserand, Robert. *Aromatherapy: To Heal and Tend the Body.* Twin Lakes: Lotus Press, 1998.

Vatsyayana. *The Complete Kama Sutra: The First Unabridged Modern Translation of the Classic Indian Text.* Translated by Alain Danielou. Rochester: Park Street Press, 1994.

Weil, Andrew, M.D. Natural Health, Natural Medicine: *A Comprehensive Manual for Wellness and Self-Care.* New York: Houghton Mifflin Company, 1998.

Zilbergeld, Bernie, Ph.D. *The New Male Sexuality.* New York: Bantam Books, 1992.